F I G H T 4 U 2

A Guide for Those With Cancer or Chronic Illness

4
Create the Ultimate Plan
2

Cheryl Merkel

Copyright

Fight4u2

ISBN: 978-1-501028-94-6
Edited by Rebecca Jaxon
Cover design and interior layout by Robin Schneider

First electronic publication: August, 2014

Praise God…

…for blessing me with this information that
I refer to as my daily bread
and the courage to share it with others.

…for His word that provided guidance and wisdom
that clearly illuminated the best path to travel,
a way that strengthened me as I faced
seemingly, insurmountable odds
with an unwavering spirit.

…for my family's unconditional love and
the encouragement of friends.

…for a caregiver with a
Kind and loving soul, that
Encourages me with a selfless, compassionate nature. His
Innovative and positive attitude uplifts me when I need it most with a
Tenderness that every person wishes for in a life partner. He embodies
Harmony and peace in the midst of chaos and uncertainty.

…for a treatment center that embraces integrated care
and the new friends I met along the way.

…for surrounding me with a village of support
that I never knew existed.

…for my work family that gave me the flexibility to
weave my career into my new life.

… and for an editor that significantly inspired me
and the development of this material.

Table of Contents

Introduction

Why Write on Limited Time?

(Then my husband reminds me, limited time is everyone's reality)

When someone loses the battle with breast cancer, oftentimes we hear the phrase, "They did everything they could for her." The word "they" in that sentence, usually referring to the doctors, is accompanied by a tone of despair. Doctors, support staff, and researchers do remarkable work for cancer patients. But since June of 2010, when I was diagnosed with Stage IV breast cancer, I learned that there are countless aspects of fighting chronic illness that complement practitioners of modern medicine.

When I was first diagnosed and still deciding where to receive treatment, there were organizations that required me to choose the traditional path (treatments that typically involve surgery, chemotherapy, and radiation) or the alternative path (treatments that strive to fight disease by naturally boosting the immune system without the use of prescription drugs or surgery) to fight cancer. Very few treatment centers embraced the idea that the two philosophies could merge and work together in harmony. Instead of following one center's approach, I took charge of my quest for wellness, and started coming up with a complementary plan to beat the odds the world was trying to dictate to me.

Not only did I learn that there were many aspects of my care that I could manage, but I also found that many cancers and other chronic illnesses, like heart disease, are what some refer to as "lifestyle diseases." If our lifestyle, spirit, and choices perhaps had a hand in this outcome, why should we not consider taking some responsibility upon ourselves to make changes that guide us back toward wellness? After my nine-month journey from stage IV breast cancer to remission, I discovered chronic illness was not necessarily a one-way street.

I envision a day when we hear "they did everything they could do for her," and the word "they" does not necessarily mean just the doctors. I prefer to hear, "She did everything she could." Replacing that one word implies a shift of empowerment from a group of professionals to one person—the patient—and the ensemble orchestrated by the patient's choices. It also uplifts the emotional tone of the phrase with an essence of perseverance, endurance, and strength.

I write this for the survivor who wants to be that person—the person who did everything possible, from a conscious decision to actively direct and participate in a personally designed plan for a better quality, and perhaps quantity, of life.

Author's Note

The purpose of this material is not to tell you step by step how to fight or prevent chronic illness; each walk is unique. It is in no way intended as a substitute for receiving medical advice or treatment. I strongly urge you to get professional opinions about your condition and to not try to self-treat your illness.

Mini Bio

I was raised in the community that the University of Illinois calls home, and my childhood and college career mirrored the experience of most of my peers. I had great friends, was active in sports, and came from a loving family who nurtured my educational plans and life goals. I played volleyball while I attended Parkland, our local community college. After graduating with honors I transferred to Northern Illinois University in DeKalb, where I received my bachelor's degree in Finance.

Within six months of graduation I started managing credit unions. My first opportunity was serving a group of members that worked at Supervalu in Urbana, Illinois. Six years passed, and I was offered the position of president of Central Illinois Credit Union in Champaign, Illinois. This is my current position and has been for nearly twenty years.

I was married for the first time in 2009 to my exceptionally supportive and positive husband. I have three sisters, and I am the stepmom to three children. They do not refer to me as their stepmom, but call me their bonus mom. Jokingly, I call myself "the bomb" for short.

I consider myself blessed, especially during the five months of intensive treatment that spanned from June to November of 2010. Not only did I work two weeks out of every three, but I stayed active by playing volleyball and walking. And I am equally grateful I remained supportive of our children's activities and church on Sundays. I didn't take up skydiving, attempt to cross things off my bucket list, or do anything crazy. I simply craved and prayed for normalcy.

Normalcy was my key objective after diagnosis. Although many of the friends I was privileged to meet through this process had varying ideas and methods of coping, one aspect remained consistent no matter what group of patients I was around. It was essential to know the story of my diagnosis before we could share anything else.

Personally, I feel the type of cancer, size of the tumor and lymph node involvement is not particularly relevant, since every case is unique. But for those who are interested, I have created a brief, yet precise, account of my diagnosis and treatment. It is a quick roadmap of my clinical journey with a splash of some accomplishments and timelines of major lifestyle changes. This personal timeline, which runs from October, 2009, to December, 2013, is located in the appendix.

Organized With a Unique Design and Format

The format of this book is inspired by the way I yearned for information shortly after diagnosis. Not only was my time limited and precious, but my decisions were tainted with a strong sense of urgency. I recall those first few weeks after my life changed. I was certainly in fight-or-flight mode. Later, when I was contemplating writing about my experiences, I had a chance to reflect on how I felt during those first few days after diagnosis. I was motivated to develop a way to share my research and experience in the simplest format possible so that you may access the information as quickly as possible.

Although I share some of my own personal stories, the majority of this information is intended to help discover your own personal path of wellness—a direction guided by your choices. I don't consider this a "how-to" book. Rather I regard it as a collection of personal experiences that improved the quality of my life. And whether that life was going to be six months or six years, I had no control over that. I felt better, and that, I did have control over.

The information is broken down into two parts. The first, a collection of the practical and physical aspects of my experience with cancer, comprises two chapters. The first chapter illustrates the choices we can control, mainly nutrition. The second chapter includes those factors that complement our food choices, such as supplementation, exercise, and alternative therapies.

The second part has a more spiritual and emotional tone, and is also divided into two chapters. The first chapter of part two reveals how I fixed my spirit from within, while the last chapter shares ideas of activities that helped me cope and adapt.

Each chapter is broken down into many different sections. I intentionally kept most of these topics short to achieve the objective of sharing a lot of material in small chunks. After you implement a lifestyle change from one of the sections, pay attention to how it impacts your energy, digestion, spirit, sleep quality, etc. Refer to the appendix and make copies of a sheet to "rate and monitor your results" to help quantify these areas within each section.

Furthermore, I realize that some prefer reading about the opinions I gathered from professionals. And others appreciate factual information, but also yearn to hear testimonies from someone who actually walked the walk. Thus, each section is broken down even more. My goal is to enable you to easily pick out the kind of information you're seeking. Before sharing an opinion, story or idea, and before quoting a fact the following keys are provided to easily identify the type of content in each section:

BC = Before Cancer: BC tells the story of the crossroads in each part of my journey. Consider them snapshots of my life that quickly and simply illustrate my starting point. Hippocrates wrote, "Illnesses do not come upon us out of the blue. They are developed from small daily sins against Nature. When enough sins have accumulated, illnesses will suddenly appear." For me to envision where I was going, I first needed to reflect on where I had been. These notes serve as a reminder that even though nothing in this book is total perfection, it is a far cry from how I treated my spirit and body in the past.

ME = My Experience: ME separates my opinion or my experience from what the experts suggest.

RE = Research Excerpts: RE signifies the quotes and paraphrased content from other authors, doctors, and experts in their field.

TRI= Tantalizing Recipes & Ideas: TRI is an opportunity for you to try the real-life examples of how I incorporated certain aspects of my new care plan into my life. My hope is to free others from some of the trial and error I engaged in myself.

WAY = Wings of Angels: WAY is the component that pulls many of these areas together. Some praise me for what I have accomplished. But because of the gift of free will from God, I still struggle to remain open to His direction. These are the stories about that relationship that blossomed when I listened.

My favorite pages are the four short stories interspersed throughout the book. They are the memoirs of my walk with God, and how His reassurance provided peace, hope and comfort. Faith gave me the encouragement that I needed—a type of encouragement that the world could not provide.

Part One
Our Bodies Are Worthy of the Best

When first diagnosed, I was bombarded by suggestions to eat certain foods like asparagus or take immune-boosting supplements such as Astragulus. These are great options for someone who is fighting cancer. But I feel fighting cancer is similar to obesity in that there is no fast track to a favorable outcome. No miracle drug or easy way to regain wellness has been developed. No endorsed product, food choice, exercise program, drug, or supplement is strong enough to stand on its own.

Likewise, living with advanced stage cancer also requires a synergistic approach, which simply means utilizing many factors that work together in harmony. I visualize plate spinners in the circus. I incorporated all these new plates into my life. I believed that if I let one slip from my attention, they may all start falling.

For instance, I know chemotherapy worked better for me because of my food choices. Supplements were effective in boosting my immune system because I was not offsetting the benefits with the toxic effects of sugar and preservatives. I cleansed my system by drinking water instead of pop and coffee. And reducing stress, walking for exercise, and finding more time for relaxation enhanced all my other lifestyle changes. In the depths of my soul, I strongly believe I would not be here if I had simply relied on chemotherapy to guide me toward remission. I am here because of many factors working together that maximized my fighting potential.

Part I is the menu of the physical changes that I tried or implemented. This collection includes sections on nutrition, supplementation, health and beauty products, and alternative therapies. While reading, take some time to reflect on your own past habits and choices, and prayerfully consider which changes could provide the best benefits for you.

"When one is diagnosed with a chronic illness and fails to change the lifestyle habits that contributed to, or perhaps caused the illness, it is like throwing gasoline on a fire."

– Mark Uram, college friend

Chapter One
The Choice is Ultimately Ours

Beware How Food is Advertised

ME

I learned that by eating out and buying food on sale, I was fueling my body with products that were provided by the lowest bidder. Sadly, price, not quality, was the driving force of my food choices.

After I began eating a healthier diet I could see the battles many Americans face every day. Not only is fast food inexpensive and abundant, but most of our grocery stores are filled with packaged foods that offer convenience and ease of preparation. These foods fit our busy lifestyles and budgets but have little or no life left in them. Processed and refined foods, usually found in the center aisles of the grocery store, are plentiful and convenient but provide limited nutritional value.

After my transition to a more natural diet, with selections rich in the foods God intended for us to eat, I realized how tempting it is to make poor food choices. It occurred to me, one Sunday, to take extra time to study the local grocery store ad. The cover of the ad highlighted 10 items that were on sale: cake mix, sugar, brown/powdered sugar, evaporated milk, chocolate chips, margarine, flour, cola, bananas, and pork butt roast.

Half of the featured items in the ad were basically processed sugar, which depresses the immune system, depletes our energy, and feeds cancer cells.

Then I thought that maybe this marketing piece did not reflect their typical advertised items. So, I picked up another copy four months later. This time on the front page they promoted the following: ham, a different kind of ham, strawberries, canned vegetables, frozen pies, canned pineapple, packaged spices, and butter.

The only advertised item still alive was the strawberries, but they are part of the Dirty Dozen, which will be explained in the next section. These ads supported my belief that making nutritional food choices does not come easy. Americans are bombarded with foods that are designed for convenience and profit, not necessarily with our best interest in mind.

BC With the hope of impressing my family, I bounded through the door proudly displaying my eighteen-inch-long cash register receipt and multiple bags of groceries totaling seventy-five dollars. I felt like such a savvy shopper, but my weekly quest for groceries had little regard for quality or nutritional value. My goal was to feed seven people for the best price possible. I placed price over quality purely from ignorance.

The Dirty Dozen

ME

Now that I have migrated to a more whole foods diet, I feel it is important to purchase organic produce whenever possible. Organic options offer the consumer a product without pesticides or fertilizers. I choose to free my body from the stress by eliminating these toxins. And I believe that by keeping my diet as pure as possible, my system can be more efficient at eliminating or controlling the disease.

RE

There are certain (nonorganic) fruits and vegetables that carry a higher pesticide load than others. The Environmental Working Group has compiled a list of these foods called, "The Dirty Dozen." By visiting their website, www.ewg.org, on a yearly basis, I keep updated on the produce highest in pesticides. The list for 2014 is as follows:

- Apples *
- Celery *
- Cherry tomatoes
- Cucumbers *
- Grapes *
- Nectarines (imported)*
- Peaches*
- Potatoes *
- Snap peas (imported)
- Spinach *
- Strawberries *
- Sweet bell peppers *

Items denoted with a (*) were also on "The Dirty Dozen" list in 2013.

Note: There are also two items not listed on the 2013 top twelve that received special mention. Although the assessment of summer squash and leafy greens did not fit into the dirty dozen criteria using the site's testing methodology, they were added as extras. They both were commonly found with pesticides that are toxic to the nervous system. In 2014 this classification included hot peppers, kale and collard greens.

Conversely, the next list of foods, called "The Clean Fifteen," has the lowest amounts of pesticides. This 2014 listing is also found at www.ewg.org/foodnews:

- Asparagus
- Avocado
- Cabbage
- Cauliflower
- Cantaloupe
- Eggplant
- Grapefruit
- Kiwi
- Mangos
- Onions
- Papayas
- Pineapples
- Sweet corn
- Sweet peas (frozen)
- Sweet potatoes

ME There are times when I buy almost everything organic, but these two lists help me prioritize when funds are tight for the week. And the information is helpful, especially during the winter, when an organic option may not be available. In the beginning of my nutritional transformation all I ate was organic produce. But these lists help me incorporate more options and variety in my diet.

TRI I made a cheat sheet by writing down the dirty dozen on one side of a card and the clean fifteen on the other. I slipped the list into a luggage tag that is clear on both sides and attached it to the handle of my purse, but it could easily be inserted into a wallet for reference.

BC I rarely ate fruits and vegetables that were raw. The minimal amount of produce I ate was usually cooked or processed with sugar and preservatives.

The Number 9

ME

In the beginning, I believed strongly that organic options were more beneficial if I was to achieve my goal for a better quality of life. But the labeling left me confused and unsure of my choices. Conventional, Natural, Greenhouse, grown in Peru? Shopping for produce was like lions and tigers and bears, oh my! I felt like I was on the yellow brick road of produce and not sure where it was going to take me.

Then I found the number 9!

When looking for organic produce, I discovered that I could cut through the marketing lingo and look for the number 9. Instead of searching for the signs on fruits and vegetables saying "organic" I could save time by simply looking at the numeric sticker on the produce. If it starts with the number nine, it is organic.

Note: While shopping for packaged foods, watch for varying levels of organic. These differences may be easily identified by the labeling, which is regulated by the U.S. Department of Agriculture. For more information visit their website, www.ams.usda.gov. Here are tips to distinguish the contents of organic products:

- **100% Organic** – All ingredients are certified organic.
- **Organic** – 95 to 99.9 percent of the ingredients are certified organic.
- **"Made with" Organic** – The product is made of at least 70 percent certified organic ingredients.
- If there are less than 70 percent certified organic ingredients, the word "organic" may not appear anywhere on the main display panel. Read the list of ingredients.

BC

I do not recall intentionally purchasing anything that was organic.

Smoothies

ME

I found it easier to consume a diet rich in fruits and vegetables by making smoothies. It is difficult for me to digest a bunch of raw produce, especially during chemotherapy, but I can drink it! Plus, I can hide less desirable ingredients like prune juice, kale and asparagus. Smoothies also give me the opportunity for more variety in my diet with less effort by just throwing different produce in the blender every day. My chiropractor recommended a Vitamix, which is a blender, rather than a juicer, which extracts just the juice from the food. He told me it is better for me to have the benefit of the whole food, including its fiber, and not just the juice.

There are supporters of juicing, like George Malkmus, the author of *The Hallelujah Diet*. But I chose to not go that route because of my chiropractor's advice. While learning to make smoothies I found raw fruits and vegetables easier to digest after they had been run through a blender. If I ate raw produce, sometimes it gave me a stomachache. There were two ways around this aside from slightly cooking the food. My first option was to chew my food until it was practically water, but that was too time-consuming. Second, I could pulverize it in the blender. This option assured me that all the produce was broken down as much as possible. It also offered insane variety and was quick. I could literally throw a salad in there with some water and organic chicken broth and drink it.

Smoothies are great because I don't need a recipe. I add produce in a blender and barely submerse it with the liquid of my choice. If it doesn't turn out that tasty, I remind myself to try and try again or drink it quicker. There have only been a few times I could not handle drinking my creation for the day. Ok, maybe more than once! But I was certainly thankful for the hundreds of tasty combinations that outweighed the less desirable ones.

As a cancer fighter, I gravitate toward berries (listed in the section on the "Top Twenty Antioxidant Foods") and green vegetables like kale and asparagus. Very seldom do I use yogurt, because I would rather eat it. Since juice is higher in sugar, I use half water and half juice as the liquid. Ice made from filtered water offers a nice substitute for water and/or juice. The ice gives my meal a different consistency, which is helpful for variety and refreshing during the summer months.

TRI As a treat, I purchase fresh-squeezed juice from the health food store. Before it reaches its expiration date, which is rather quick at times, I pour the remaining juice into ice cube trays and used them for my smoothies.

Bananas also freeze well once peeled. By breaking them in pieces before storing in a freezer bags, I can easily utilize them when needed.

It is also beneficial to purchase blueberries in bulk. I buy them from a local farm ten pounds at a time. Then I wash them, put the berries on a towel to fully dry and pack them in freezer bags.

One of my favorite combinations for smoothies is:

- 4-6 frozen strawberries
- ½ cup of frozen blueberries
- ½ frozen banana
- ½ cup of frozen raspberries, cherries or pineapple
- 1 ½ cup of liquid (I use ¾ cup of organic or fresh squeezed juice and ¾ cup filtered water)
- (Optional) 4-6 ounces of plain organic yogurt. Plain, organic Greek yogurt, which is high in protein, is a great option.
- (Optional) 2-3 frozen orange juice cubes from an ice cube tray or ice cubes made from filtered water to make the meal thicker.
- (Optional) 1 cup of kale, spinach or romaine. I grew to appreciate adding vegetables to my recipes over time. When I was new to this, however, I favored fruit, yogurt, and juice.

BC I recall enjoying smoothies on occasion and feeling great after drinking them, but I was too absorbed in the hustle and bustle of life to incorporate them into my daily routine. Nor did I take the time to truly embrace how different they made me feel. And believe me, one little smoothie did not have a chance of compensating for the hundreds of worthless foods I put in my body at that time.

Free-Range Meat

ME

My nutritionist told me that if money was tight, it was more important to purchase free-range, grass-fed meat, than to use my budget for organic produce, because this option provided a product without antibiotics or hormones. She also advised me to purchase wild-caught fish rather than farm-raised. She said I could wash most of the unnatural additives off produce, but I couldn't do the same with meat and fish. So, good quality meat was usually my first priority.

I had sticker shock when I paid ten to thirty dollars a pound for meat and fish. But I found that as I migrated more and more to a whole foods diet, I craved less meat. Not only did I eat it less frequently, but I also ate less at each meal. A pound of lean meat stretched out over multiple servings.

RE

In George Malkmus's book, *The Hallelujah Diet,* he compares how meat impacts our bodies now in relation to biblical times. "Animal products are currently the cause of up to 90 percent of all physical problems experienced by people. The average person who consumes animal products puts into their body some 100 pounds of fat in one year. Back in Bible days, meat contained roughly three percent fat. Today, beef is 20 to 40 percent fat, because of modern grain-feeding techniques. Pork is 40 to 60 percent fat. A chicken breast today, even if you remove the skin and broil it, still has a very high fat content."

I used to wonder why God did not intend for us to eat pork. I thought it was the other white meat! Indeed God was telling us what to do, but He was also protecting us because pork has a high fat content.

Note: There are free-range pork products, but I choose not to eat them.

BC

I thought meat was meat. I did not know there was an option such as grass-fed, free-range meat and poultry.

Protein Sources Other Than Meat

In the book *The Hallelujah Diet* this sentence jumped out at me from the pages: "There's evidence linking a high meat diet to Alzheimer's disease and breast cancer." That got my attention. My life BC, before cancer, was rich in meat consumption. I know I ate more meat than grains, fruits, and vegetables at times. Especially during my high-protein-diet days, when I valued weight loss over wellness.

At first, it was hard for me to make the transition from meat- to plant-based proteins. Then I read *The China Study,* by Dr. T. Colin Campbell, and the adjustment didn't seem quite as challenging. Dr. Campbell theorizes that most American diseases are caused by meat and dairy. I recommend reading The China Study, if you are fighting a chronic illness like cancer or heart disease.

I limited my meat, but I didn't cut it out of my diet completely. My cancer fighter team had suggested a goal of 70 grams of protein per day for healing. Whenever I needed a boost, I still ate chicken or fish. A four-ounce serving of chicken has 30 grams. But to balance my nutritionist's plea for protein in my diet and my desire to cut down meat consumption, I turned to nutritional labels. I also found protein in:

Oatmeal	7 g
Yogurt (8 oz) *Greek yogurt can be higher*	10 g
Nuts (1/4 cup pumpkin or sunflower)	9 g
Almonds (3 tablespoons)	6 g
Beans (1/2 cup cooked pinto, black, lentil)	5-8 g
One egg	6 g
Cottage cheese (4 oz)	13 g

My interest was piqued the day my chiropractor reminded me I could get protein and calcium from green leafy vegetables. Then I read the following passage from *The Hallelujah Diet:* "If there is protein in the flesh of an animal, then where did all that protein come from? It came directly from the grass it ate! If there's calcium in the cow's milk, where did all that calcium come from? The grass! All the nutrients in an animal first came through the raw vegetation it ate. And when you eat the animal, you are getting the nutrients secondhand." Later in the book he added, "Furthermore, animal products do not contain phytochemicals, flavonoids and antioxidants. These nutrients boost the immune system with the ability to fight cancer and heart disease." So after listening to George Malkmus and my chiropractor, I decided to try to gain some of my protein straight from the source by eating green leafy vegetables instead of so much meat.

Another huge supporter of plant-based protein is, Alissa Cohen, the author of *Raw Foods for Everyone*. Here is her stand on the animal- versus plant-based-protein debate. "Foods that we often think of as the best sources of protein—beef, chicken, fish and eggs—do not create protein in your body. Amino acids create protein in your body. And the best source of amino acids is leafy green vegetables such as spinach, kale and chard." She gives an example of the protein in a chicken breast. A chicken breast starts with about 20 grams of protein until it is cooked and that amount is cut in half. Then once this 10 grams is consumed it can take about one hundred hours for your body to fully process it. Throughout all this processing you may have absorbed a couple grams of protein. On the other hand greens and sprouts start with fewer grams of protein, but your body will benefit from almost all the raw food has to offer. Plus, it is less taxing on your system because it is easier to process than animal protein. One other benefit is that plant-based protein does not have the risk of passing on hormones that meat does.

ME

After making the switch from lean meats to plant-based proteins my energy level increased. I now know that if I eat meat, my productivity and zest for life suffers. I have become more aware of how my food choices impact my quality of life.

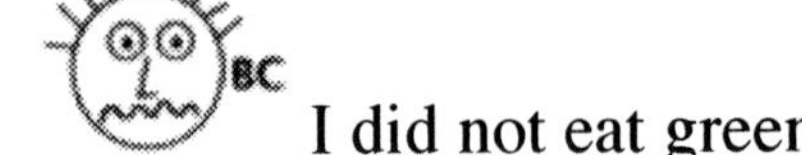

I did not eat green, leafy vegetables, usually just traditional head lettuce.

Foods That God Intended For Us to Eat

ME WAY Days after diagnosis, while I was at the Christian book store searching for a Bible, I found on the top shelf of an adjacent section a book by Jordan Rubin called *The Maker's Diet*. My thoughts were immediately drawn to this book as if an angel's light were shining down on that section of the store to get my attention. My primary care physician had suggested *The Maker's Diet* to me months earlier at my yearly physical. For some reason I vividly remembered that conversation and decided to pick up Jordan Rubin's book along with my first devotional Bible.

I have always struggled with weight, because I find comfort in eating. So, I was moved to give the diet a try. From the conversation with my doctor months earlier and the title of the book, it seemed as if this material offered more than just a food plan. Jordan Rubin illustrated how proper nutrition can facilitate healing. He personally struggled with chronic health problems that western and eastern medicine could not cure. He literally traveled the world to search for answers. After all options were exhausted, he ended up finding his own cure by means of proper nutrition.

Rubin developed a diet based on the foods that God intended for us to eat. It is a three-phase plan that spans over forty days. The first two-week phase is rich in foods like berries, nuts, lean meats, fish, and vegetables. Fortunately, I was able to follow Rubin's recommended plan for a little over a month before my chemotherapy started, and I truly believe it detoxified and strengthened my body to the "best me" I could be before starting chemotherapy. I almost felt invincible going into treatment. It was actually the best I had felt in years, even though two of my major organs, my liver and my lungs, were full of cancer. And not only did I feel great before treatment started, but I also remained active during chemotherapy.

From that gift of proper nutrition, my interests spun off in other directions, which I will discuss in later sections. I do want to stress that since I began following *The Maker's Diet,* I have not changed the foundational principles of what I eat. I still eat mostly organic, whole foods, and I feel better now than I had felt in a long time.

ME Not only did I learn about the power of proper nutrition weeks before my chemotherapy started in 2010, but I also shared this experience with my husband during Lent of 2013. As a couple we implemented the forty-day, three-phase program as an internal cleansing.

We both struggle with weight and although my diet had changed and I had incorporated many of these foods into my lifestyle, he was still eating the Standard American Diet. This time I recorded all the changes we recognized. When I followed *The Maker's Diet* in 2010 I knew I felt incredible, I just did not take the time to notice all the little changes. This time it was fun to discover the positive differences together.

This is our personal list from our experience with *The Maker's Diet*:

- insane energy
- brighter eyes
- clearer skin
- clearer heads (thoughts and communication came easier)
- pain-free knees (especially on stairs)
- better sleep (quality was increased rather than quantity)
- refreshed feeling in the morning (woke most of the time without an alarm)
- decreased gas and bloating (One morning we woke up and were reflecting on the changes and my husband blurted out, "I never fart anymore!")
- reduced snoring
- quiet mind (My shiatsu therapist calls a racing mind, "monkey mind." I find I can control these random, usually meaningless thoughts better with proper nutrition.)
- calm body (Both my husband and I had restless legs in the evening. Sometimes it was difficult for us to sit still, especially when we ate dairy.)
- pleasant mood (The kids said that Dad seemed nicer. This was my personal favorite.)

All these changes decreased our stress and increased our positive attitude and zest for life.

BC I didn't even realize there were so many foods listed in the Bible that should and should not be eaten.

Foods Compatible with Blood Type

RE Dr. Peter J. D'Adamo wrote the book *Live Right 4 Your Type*. He analyzed how people process food differently based on their blood type. I have Type A blood, which, according to Dr. D'Adamo, made me more prone to cancer, heart disease, and diabetes than any other blood type. Yay for me! This information did help reinforce the importance of diet.

ME

Since reading his book, I very, very rarely eat wheat, dairy, red meat, or potatoes. Keep in mind, these are the foods I avoid because of my blood type. Some blood types flourish on meat and do not do well with most grains. And there are some people who do not process chicken well. The diet is tailored for each blood type. And when I follow it, I feel better.

Because of the changes I made, food does not bog me down anymore or upset my stomach. This diet, along with *The Maker's Diet* in the previous section, created the foundation of my food choices today.

TRI Wheat was the hardest food for me to give up. I found a great alternative with spelt. I buy spelt bread, pretzels, crackers and tortilla shells. To my surprise spelt tastes closer to white bread than whole wheat, and I prefer these options over the traditional ones. As a bonus they do not bloat or upset my stomach.

I used to love sour cream! But I found that I did not process dairy well either. Since plain yogurt is fermented, it does not tax my digestive system, and it serves as a great alternative. When I use it on tacos, it really does not taste that different than sour cream. And I actually prefer it.

Last but not least was salad dressing. I dreadfully missed commercial salad dressing. I ate salad with olive oil, for about a year, but found it pretty boring. Then I discovered a flavor explosion when I squeezed lime juice over the salad with the olive oil.

There are some yogurt-based salad dressings, made with natural ingredients, on the market that I enjoy on occasion. Some of them do not have dairy, but I watch the vinegar content, which is not compatible with my blood type. Therefore, when I have time, I like to make my own dressing in the blender.

Salad Dressing

- plain organic yogurt or greek yogurt (4 parts)
- organic salsa (2 parts)
- avocado (2 parts)
- sea salt (to taste)
- lime (to taste)
- Note: for a zestier taste use equal parts yogurt, salsa and avocado

ME

The possible correlation between food and blood type were reinforced during a conversation with a fellow cancer survivor. In our first meeting we really hit it off. I knew she researched cancer and nutrition when I learned that she had Type O blood. I waited in anticipation of where this conversation was going. She told me that she had switched to a vegan diet about ten years earlier. (According to Dr. D'Adamo people with Type O blood thrive as meat eaters.) When she had made this switch, she felt terrible. She also believed that stressors, like this change in diet, could possibly have planted the seed that developed into cancer later in life.

This conversation allowed me to reflect on my own possible nutritional stressor. About ten years before my diagnosis I followed a strict protein diet for about one year. I ate mostly animal proteins, but remember, I have Type A blood. And Type As thrive as vegetarians. We both had good intentions, but did we possibly stress our bodies out by the food choices we made? Unfortunately, sometimes we learn the rules in life after the game has already started.

Note: Throughout this compilation of material I focused on Type A blood because that was my type, along with 40 percent of the population. For more information on Type A blood and the effect of other blood types on food choices visit his website, www.dadamo.com, or read *Live Right 4 Your Type*, by Dr. D'Adamo. Don't know your blood type? Blood typing test kits may be purchased at health food stores.

BC

Looking back I assumed I was healthy as I migrated to a high protein diet, with no regard for fat content, because I lost weight easily. When I was young, I associated weight loss with wellness. During this time I ate lots of fast food hamburgers with extra condiments and no bun. I loved fajitas with extra sour cream and no shells. But my diet was devoid of fruits, vegetables, nuts, and whole grains, which in hindsight may have been a poor choice for me.

Manage the Sugar Addiction

ME

I have been told more than once that sugar, stress, and unresolved emotional issues are some of the underlying factors that may increase the risk of cancer. Regaining control of sugar may have been imperative, a necessary change for remission.

Of course, I questioned everything I heard and read, and I wondered whether sugar had anything to do with cancer growth. Then I thought about the injection they put in the blood stream for PET scans. They ask patients to fast before a PET scan because they inject them with radioactive *sugar*. This injection goes right to the cancerous growth. Cancer feeds on sugar! Because that patient has fasted for six hours, the radioactive sugar lights up the tumors on the scan and shows the doctors where the cancer is located. Not only does cancer like sugar, but it also, according to my chiropractor, depresses the immune system. By consuming it, I was crippling my body's ability to fight.

After I freed myself from sugar, I still struggled with a dependence that I compared to some prescription or street drugs. Not only was sugar addictive for me and still is, but the more I ate, the more I needed, because I became immune to the effects of the sugar. In other words, the more I ate, the less I felt the reward. And I ate more to achieve the same satisfaction. Sounds like an addictive drug to me!

RE

According to George Malkmus, author of *The Hallelujah Diet*, in the last one hundred years, sugar consumption has grown from an average of 5 to 170 pounds per year. It is crazy to think some eat their weight in sugar every year. Also, cancer is not picky. It loves sugar in all its forms. So, now I also watch for ingredients like high fructose corn syrup and white flour too.

History proves humans have had an amazing track record of adapting to change, but not that quickly. One hundred years is not enough time to adjust to an extra 165 pounds of sugar.

BC

I ate whatever sugar, natural or artificial, that I could get my hands on!

No Hormones and No Hot Flashes

ME

Believe it or not, I did not suffer from hot flashes! I thought it was just good luck. Lupron, the drug administered every three months to suppress the activity of my ovaries, and chemotherapy should have pushed me into menopause. But I was amazed to find that somehow I had avoided them. I had hot flashes before I was diagnosed. So, I knew what they felt like. I expected something worse, but all of a sudden, the symptoms were gone!

Then I thought that maybe I was already premenopausal before treatment, and that the chemotherapy pushed me through on the express route. But the hot flashes came back a couple weeks after I stopped the Maker's Diet. During this forty-day program, I had avoided dairy and high-fat meats. I had incorporated mozzarella cheese back into my diet after migrating from the Maker's Diet, and I realized that was the difference. What a gift! I realized, on my own, how food affected my body, even its effect on hot flashes. I later discovered all dairy (except yogurt), red meat, and wine made flare ups for me.

Some of the foods I can still eat are chicken, turkey, fish, yogurt, and rice/almond milk. I recommend to others who suffer from hot flashes to keep a food log. This will more than likely help pinpoint what foods aggravate the problem.

Of course, my next concern was the amount of calcium I was receiving without dairy in my diet. My chiropractor assured me that I could get the calcium I needed from organic rice/almond milk, yogurt, and green leafy vegetables. But calcium is especially important after chemotherapy, so I also take a calcium supplement.

Note on dairy: Watch nutritional labels. Dairy may be found in other products, like taco seasoning. I am not picking on taco seasoning, but it serves as a reminder that dairy may exist in foods that might come as a surprise. When I remind people who have hot flashes to watch their dairy, the first response is "Oh, I do not drink milk." Dairy is way more than milk. If I have even a little dairy, I get hot flashes. It is certainly worth the sacrifice to avoid it for a couple of days to see if it makes a difference.

BC

I suffered miserably from hot flashes. They were so bad that our mattress pad had mold spots underneath the area where I slept from all the moisture.

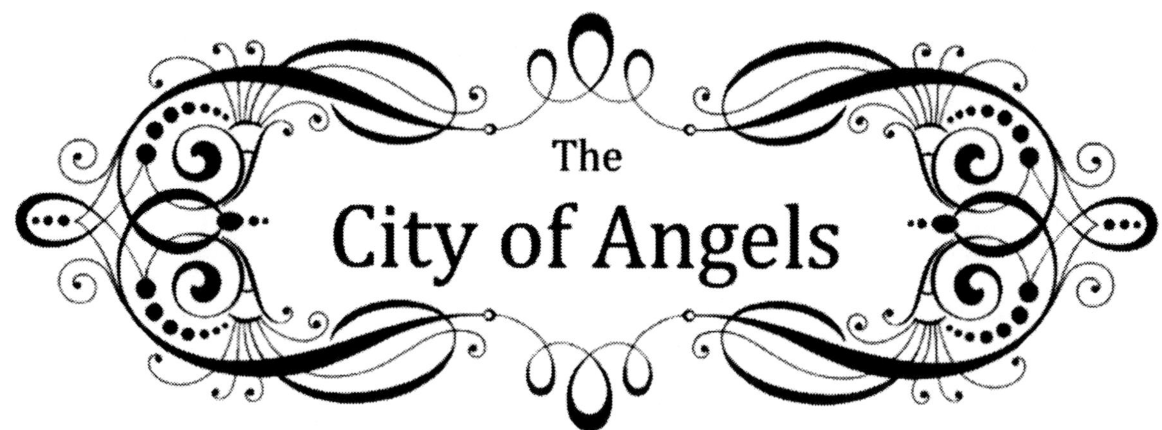

Where to go for treatment? What an overwhelming decision at such an indecisive time in my life. A Stage IV diagnosis was terrifying, and when I combined that feeling with the knowledge that the decisions I was about to make—about my chemotherapy regimen, and about where to go for it—could give me my best shot of beating cancer, it was a lot to take in. During this time, which was after surgery and before chemotherapy started, I had received a couple of cards from the babysitter who had cared for me as a child. She closed every note by saying "Remember the Angels." This phrase brought me comfort. But also, after multiple such notes from her, I could not help but take notice.

Days later, my husband came home with a business card. On the back was a phone number. Above the number was the phrase "City of Angels." He had a friend who had gone to Cancer Treatment Centers of America (CTCA). His friend's family called CTCA the "City of Angels" because of the exceptional care and compassion he received. So I called them a couple days later believing all these angel references were a sign that could not be ignored. Once I made the call, they took care of all my arrangements, and I was set to go.

My sister reinforced my decision later that day when she told me she was doing research about CTCA and minutes later one of her co-workers came into her office. He told her how his mother was treated there and of the positive experience she had, just like the treatment my husband's friend received.

All these coincidences happened within days of each other. I look back on it now and realize it was God working through others to guide me. If I had stayed in my hometown, the testing and results were estimated to take much longer. Plus, the local doctor wanted to biopsy my liver, which CTCA did not recommend. I was more comfortable with that.

Ultimately, I went where I felt content, especially after I reflected on the coincidences that got me there. There was no doubt in my mind that Cancer Treatment Centers of America was where I was supposed to be.

But the coincidences did not stop once I made the choice to be treated at the integrated-care cancer center in Zion, Illinois. I had all the scans and appointments with the intake doctors to determine our course of action, and it was time for me to meet with the oncologist. As I waited in the room the nurse informed me that my oncologist was on vacation, and someone else would be filling in for her. She assured me that I was in great hands and that he was a retired doctor who had flown in to be there for the patients. I remembered feeling a little deflated, but as soon as he walked in the door, that all melted away.

Even though my dad, who was with me at the time, is not one who is easily flustered, and even while I was in the midst of a Stage IV cancer diagnosis, I saw the anxiety lift from his shoulders as soon as the doctor started his examination. His experienced techniques of reading my body were intriguing to me. At one point I remember him thumping my abdomen like a watermelon—almost as if he could read the tumor by the sound that resonated from my belly. He wrote three chemotherapy drugs on a little piece of white paper and told me that these were the drugs that he recommended.

I left there thinking my life is surely in God's hands, but is this where I am supposed to be? I was exhausted from questioning every decision. So, I looked to others for guidance. My parents and husband joined me for the initial consultation, and they were all comfortable with the doctor and his confidence in my treatment plan and compassionate nature. That evening I had my first treatment. I crawled into bed at eleven o'clock, relieved that the final decision had been made and the implementation begun.

Three weeks after my first ever chemotherapy treatment, and now bald, I met my permanent oncologist. Not only was she pleased to share the unbelievable results, since my blood work revealed my tumor markers were within the normal range. But she also apologized to me and my family for not being present at the first visit. I told her that everyone needs a vacation and how much we enjoyed meeting her replacement. Of course, I had to ask whether she would have chosen the same course of treatment that the other doctor had begun. She said that this was not exactly what she would have recommended, but close. But why change it, since it seemed to work rather effectively!

Could it all be a coincidence? Starting with the card that said, "Remember the Angels," to meeting an oncologist who seemed to be an angel sent from heaven to recommend the best chemotherapy plan for me. I still sit and marvel at the chain of events and now realize God was orchestrating His plan.

Top Twenty Antioxidant Foods

RE A listing on About.com of a study conducted by the U.S. Department of Agriculture measured the antioxidant levels of foods commonly eaten by Americans. The top twenty foods are:

Food	Portion	Antioxidant Level
Red Beans (dried)	½ cup	13,727
Wild Blueberries	1 cup	13,427
Red Kidney Beans (dried)	½ cup	13,259
Pinto Beans	½ cup	11,864
Blueberries	1 cup	9,019
Whole Cranberries	1 cup	8,983
Artichokes (cooked)	1 cup	7,904
Blackberries	1 cup	7,701
Prunes	½ cup	7,291
Raspberries	1 cup	6,085
Strawberries	1 cup	5,938
Red Delicious Apples	1	5,900
Granny Smith Apples	1	5,381
Pecans	1 ounce	5,095
Cherries	1 cup	4,873
Black Plums	1	4,844
Russet Potatoes (cooked)	1	4,649
Black Beans (dried)	½ cup	4,181
Red Plums	1	4,118
Gala Apples	1	3,903

TRI

The hardest nutritional obstacle for me to reinvent was snacks. I learned to incorporate some of these foods not only into my meals but some of my munchies too.

Apples with some kind of nut butter or raw honey is a convenient on the go food. My favorite raw honey product is a cinnamon infused product by YS Eco Bee Farms called CINNA Honey Raw, which is also great with strawberries.

I also use the CINNA Honey by placing a teaspoon along the edge of a bowl. I dislike washing dishes. So, I use the same teaspoon to scoop out 4-5 spoonfuls of plain organic yogurt. I top the yogurt with blueberries, raspberries or blackberries. I incorporate some more Omega-3s in my diet by squeezing some flax seed oil or spreading ground flax seed over everything. I eat this snack by taking a portion of the honey from the side of the bowl and then scooping up the rest of the contents in the bowl. It can all be stirred together, but I enjoy eating it in proportions of my choice.

BC

I only ate three foods from the antioxidant list. One was potatoes, which are not compatible with my blood type. And I am not sure if refried beans at the Mexican restaurant qualify as a serving of pinto beans. If it does, then that was my second. The third was apples, but I only ate non-organic Gala apples, and only on occasion.

Foods Contain Estrogen?

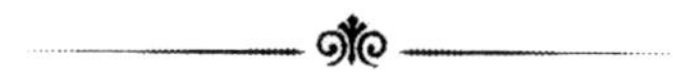

RE

As a breast cancer survivor, I was aware that tumor growth could be receptive to hormones. But I was surprised to find out that hormones were also found in the foods I ate. Not only were there foods that added to my estrogen load, but there were also choices that could help reduce it. There is a website, www.holisticonline.com, that breaks these foods down into two groups: foods that naturally contain estrogen and foods that help inhibit it.

Note: Some of the more common estrogen rich foods are apples, animal flesh, carrots, cherries, cucumbers, dairy, eggs, oats, olive oil, peas, potatoes, rice, soybeans, sunflower seeds, tomatoes, and wheat.

ME

Even though I had tumors that responded to estrogen, I did not stop eating estrogen-rich foods. However, I was conscious of my food choices. For instance, if I was faced with eating an apple or berries, I picked the berries most of the time. I still ate antioxidant-rich apples on occasion, just not every day. After reflecting on my dietary choices I realized I had been eating too much estrogen-rich foods and not enough of the foods that swept it away.

The topic of soy products leaves many survivors confused. Initially, I didn't receive a clear-cut answer on soy from dieticians either. But even if soy had the potential to add more to my estrogen load, I was intrigued after I read about women from other countries that eat soy all the time and have very little breast cancer. I decided to compromise by limiting my soy to no more than one serving per day. I want to stress that this is my opinion. I simply decided to go with the view that most choices are good in moderation. My soy consumption is limited to occasionally having some edamame, soy milk when I do not have access to rice milk, and some miso broth mixed with filtered water for more flavor when I cook brown rice.

Since my diagnosis in 2010, there has been more and more research on breast cancer and soy. Websites such as PubMed, www.pubmed.gov, have published more recent studies on the benefits of soy that is naturally found in foods and breast cancer. This website is a great resource for keeping up to date on the latest research.

BC I ate an abundance of estrogen-rich foods like meat, dairy, eggs, and wheat, but I rarely consumed foods that swept it away.

Cancer Prefers an Acidic Environment

ME RE I am sure that all the choices I outlined in the previous sections make the task of keeping everything in balance resemble a juggling act. I promise this is the last nutritional factor to consider.

There are foods that are alkalizing and foods that are acidic. Since acidic diets promote inflammation, most wellness diets promote eating more *alkaline* foods, which mainly consists of fruits and vegetables. When I plan my meals, at a minimum I strive to match alkaline foods with acidic options. For example if I have a piece of lean meat, I try to eat a vegetable with it instead of rice or bread. Or if I eat free range eggs for breakfast, I have a side of blueberries. So, for every serving of acidic food I try to balance the pH in my body with a serving of alkaline food. According to Don Colbert, MD, the author of *The Seven Pillars of Health*, the "alkaline-forming foods include most fruits, green vegetables, lentils, spices, herbs and seasonings, and seeds and nuts. Acid-forming foods include meat, fish, poultry, chicken eggs, most grains, legumes, and especially desserts, processed foods, and fast foods." There is also detailed information about these foods at the Acid Alkaline Diet website, www.acidalkalinediet.com, or at Essence of Life, www.essence-of-life.com.

ME I use test strips that are available over the counter at most health food stores to monitor pH levels. On occasion I test my urine first thing in the morning to check my system's pH. I perform the test in the mornings, because I have found that food and exercise have a temporary impact on the results. I urinate on the tip of the strip. Then I immediately determine the results by matching it to the color chart on the box and discard the soiled strip in the toilet. It is very quick and simple.

An easy way to adjust pH to higher alkaline levels is to do a one day fruit/vegetable juice fast. Another quick way to raise pH is to try lemon or lime juice squeezed into drinking water.

Note: Don't freak out! I found my pH to be low, which means my system was more acidic, after chemotherapy treatments. Prescription drugs also made my pH acidic; I attempted to balance it out by taking my magnesium supplement, which is more alkaline than acidic, with them.

Coffee is known to be an antioxidant. For the first year after diagnosis, all I had to drink was water, green tea and occasionally juice. Once I was in remission for a couple months, I thought I could incorporate coffee into my diet again. I actually missed coffee more than pop, and I had been a huge pop drinker. So, I tried it for a couple of weeks. I could not get my pH in balance, since coffee is extremely acidic. My knees started hurting; acidity promotes inflammation. I was not sleeping well at night. The most alarming change was that my eczema was showing signs of flaring up again. I dropped coffee out of my diet, and all was well again. That test further proved that I continually needed to listen to my body and nourish it with foods that enhanced my life.

BC

My diet consisted mostly of eggs, corn, grains, dairy, meat, sugar, coffee and soft drinks. Since I mixed diet and regular cola at the soda fountain, my soft drinks were high in multiple kinds of sweeteners and were extremely acidic.

One Master List

ME

To keep all the information from the previous sections straight I compiled the foods into one master list. Since the blood-type diet is specialized for my system, I began with those foods as the starting point (see the section "Foods Compatible with Blood Type" for more information). On the copied pages from the blood-type diet I put E+ or E- by each food to remind me which foods add estrogen and which swept it away. Then I put an Ak by the alkaline foods and Ac by the Acidic Foods. I also noted which foods I should buy organic. Next, I put a star by the top twenty antioxidant foods. Finally, I narrowed all these choices down to those that were listed in the Bible and *The Maker's Diet* by Jordan Rubin. So, I crossed out foods like pork, shell fish, and catfish, the unclean meats. This list provided great direction while I shopped, but I became curious. Which foods were the best? Which foods had the most beneficial properties? I listed the foods on a handmade spreadsheet and started making check marks beside them to indicate blood-type compatibility, alkalinity, antioxidant value, and estrogen.

I am proud to share "Cheryl's List of Super Foods." The foods on this first list are beneficial for my blood type, they are alkaline, some of the choices are rich in antioxidants, and none of them naturally produce high amounts of estrogen. This list consists of the foods I eat as much as possible:

- Blackberry (organic)
- Lime
- Pineapple
- Celery (organic)
- Onion
- Parsley
- Kale (organic)

This next list includes foods that are not "super" beneficial for me according to the blood-type diet, but are still beneficial or at worst, neutral, nonetheless. Most of them are alkaline. Some of these foods are good for preparing with more acidic food choices. Some naturally contain estrogen. This list includes:

Blueberry (organic)	Cherry	Lemon	Pineapple Juice
Soy sauce	Green tea	Asparagus	Raspberries
Strawberry (organic)	Cantaloupe	Kiwi	Watermelon
Sea Salt	Olive oil	Flaxseed	Green beans
Lentils	Pinto beans	Broccoli	Carrot
Romaine (organic)	Garlic	Cinnamon	Avocado
Oatmeal	Zucchini	Almonds	Pumpkin seeds
Ginger	Miso		

Important Reminder: Keep in mind this is my list of foods. I am not suggesting that you eat more of these foods too. I simply share this list to illustrate that it's possible to come up with a list of power foods to help fight or prevent disease. But I am pretty confident if you are a triple-positive breast cancer survivor (meaning the tumor is responsive to estrogen, progesterone and HER2) with Type A blood, this list may be as helpful to you as it was for me.

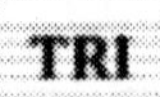

Crock-Pot Oatmeal

For my busy lifestyle, a great breakfast that includes a lot of these foods into my diet is crock-pot oatmeal. I take 2 cups of steel cut oatmeal and mix it with 6 cups of liquid (½ filtered water and ½ rice milk). I cook it on low in the crock-pot for about 4 hours. I prefer oatmeal more on the thick side than runny, but the amount of liquid used determines the consistency. I keep the leftover oatmeal in the refrigerator for breakfast throughout the work week. In the morning I heat it up on the stove and add cinnamon, almonds, ground flaxseed, organic blueberries, and raw honey.

Power Pasta (great for a quick dinner)

- Cook noodles as directed on the label (I prefer Soba or Kamut).
- Add olive oil and sea salt to the cooked and strained noodles to taste.
- Then add some beneficial foods. Here is what I use:
  - o Romaine and/or spinach
  - o Shredded carrots
  - o Shredded zucchini
  - o Avocado chunks
  - o Pumpkin seeds
  - o Lime juice squeezed over everything to taste

BC

I ate some of these foods, but only on occasion. In the past I considered eating most of these foods as a sacrifice rather than a gift.

Not a Purist

ME

Throughout my treatment, I was diligent about my dietary choices most of the time. I made some discoveries along the way that worked for me even though they were not part of the Cheryl-super-foods plan. One of my favorite treats was a muffin from our local health food store and a fruit smoothie. I felt energized when I had this for breakfast. For some, the muffin may have bogged them down, but it made me feel great. Even though white flour is a cancer-fighting no-no, it got me through chemotherapy. After researching nutrition I came up with these possible feel-good reasons:

- The acid of the muffin is neutralized by the alkalizing effect of the fruit in the smoothie.
- The white flour sweeps away estrogen; whole wheat increases the estrogen load.
- Since both items are made at the health food store, all the ingredients are natural or organic without added ingredients or preservatives.
- Strawberries are high in vitamin C, and the blueberries are high in antioxidants.

I still appreciate this for breakfast before my morning walk. Most importantly, I enjoy it! Is white flour and sugar good for fighting cancer? No, it probably is not the best choice, but I feel good. Once I changed my eating habits, I became more sensitive to what I call "instinctual eating." Just like our household pets eat instinctually, I am aware of what makes me thrive and what depletes my energy.

Oftentimes people ask how I coped with avoiding or limiting certain foods. For me, one such food was pizza. I loved it, but it didn't love me. When I ate it, my energy was zapped, my digestion came to a standstill, and I became bloated. I managed the craving by reframing the situation as a choice rather than a sacrifice. Think of it this way. Telling myself "I choose not to eat pizza" was much easier for me to accept than "I can never eat pizza again." Rather than dwelling on what I couldn't have, I embraced that I was in control of empowering choices.

BC

A typical meal before I was diagnosed made me want to take a nap. But now if I eat right, I can go, go, go with pleasure and abundant energy.

What Are Enzymes?

ME

Growing up I admired the longevity of my mother's side of the family. They experienced active lifestyles well into their eighties. I assumed the secret of their long lives was the work and love they put into their gardening hobby, as it gave them more purpose in their golden years. Being active most of my life I assumed that gardening provided exercise, which may have been a contributing factor, but now I realize that it was because their food was bursting with enzymes. That was the key. The food they ate added quality years to their life because they consumed produce that was alive, and life creates life.

RE

Ok, so what is an enzyme? Webster's dictionary defines enzymes as "any of the various protein-like substances, formed in plant and animal cells, that act as organic catalysts in initiating or speeding up specific chemical reactions and that usually become inactive or unstable at high temperatures."

The Enzyme Factor, by Dr. Hiromi Shinya, was a great resource for understanding the power of enzymes. His theory is that we are born with a certain amount of enzymes, and when this supply is depleted, illness and then death is the result. So, just as we refuel our cars with gasoline, we must replenish our bodies with enzymes. The easiest way to accomplish this is by eating raw foods.

Not only does a poor diet increase the risk of depleting our enzymes, but free radicals also compromise these reserves. Dr. Shinya documented pollution, stress, preservatives, smoking, alcohol, and electromagnetic/ultraviolet rays as factors that accelerate the extinction of these vital life forces.

His theory of this God-given enzyme reserve also explains why all of us can eat the Standard American Diet for a certain period of time, and then our bodies start to break down. When the supply gets low, we have mild symptoms such as fatigue, headaches, and digestive issues. Then when the supply becomes depleted, illness sets in.

Of course, I can't help but think about the people who live full lives while smoking, drinking, and eating meals passed through a drive-through window. It usually comes down to attitude. They are the happy-go-lucky people who manage stress well. Dr. Shinya reinforces this in his book too. He says that we can boost our enzymes simply by genuine feelings of love, gratitude, and worthwhile goals, while our feelings of loneliness and negativity, along with all the other daily sins committed against our body, destroy enzymes.

I decided that if there was a possibility my life could be cut short simply because I wasted my God-given, precious reserves of enzymes, then I should pick a lifestyle that allowed me to restore them.

TRI Produce management was foreign to me. In the beginning I wasted a lot of food because I didn't know how to store or prepare it. After much experimentation, here are some of my favorite tips:

- Apples are best refrigerated. I thought they looked good in a bowl on the kitchen table, but they do not last as long.
- Strawberries stay fresh longer if they are stored without cleaning them first.
- Grapes can be frozen for a refreshing treat, especially in the hotter months.
- Greens should be stored unwashed and then rinsed well before use. I love the plastic bags or containers designed for produce storage.
- Greens, such as Swiss chard, make a great replacement for tortilla shells.
- A couple hours before eating a pineapple I cut off the crown, the end that the leafy greens come out of, and place the pineapple upside down on a plate and store it in the fridge. The juices run from the bottom throughout the entire piece of fruit before I cut it up and serve it.
- To get the maximum amount of juice, I firmly roll whole limes or lemons under my hand before I cut them.

From SAD to RAW

ME

I had never eaten raw zucchini in my entire life. I usually refrain from using the word never, but I truly do not recall the experience before cancer. So, the fact that I eat it now and actually enjoy it is a miracle. I learned to eat food like this by what I call food combining or matching, or by many ingredients layered together in one dish—as my aunt puts it, "pile-on."

When I was learning to embrace a whole-foods diet, initially I thought it implied that I had to eat raw vegetables, period. The thought of sitting down to a bowl of lettuce and a side of raw carrots after growing up on the Standard American Diet was not my idea of how to end my work day. I used to reward myself with food, and now I felt as if meals were a punishment. Nevertheless, I knew I had to change. Somehow I needed to find a way to eat foods that were alive, not processed.

By matching fruits and vegetables with other foods, I learned to appreciate the flavor and the energy raw foods provided. There were times when I yearned to eat what my friends did when we went out for dinner. But for the most part, I preferred the new palette not only for the taste, but for how I felt after the meal.

TRI

Since zucchini is mentioned in the beginning of this section, I include it here in my first example. All the ingredients may be adjusted to taste. These amounts are listed as a guideline.

Lucky 7 Layer Salad

- 1 cup of shredded zucchini on the bottom of a bowl
- 4T plain organic yogurt – enough to cover the zucchini
- 3T salsa
- ½ cup cooked ground turkey or chicken
- ½ medium diced onion – sautéed with coconut oil and the poultry
- A Tablespoon of ground flax seed
- Sprinkle with pumpkin or sunflower seeds

(For more flavor add sea salt or fresh squeezed lime juice to taste)

I even utilize the food combining concept into my breakfast, which was and still is my favorite meal of the day. Before diagnosis, I ate a bagel with one scrambled egg almost every day of the week. I had a hard time switching to eggs without meat and bread until I started making the following recipe.

Egg Salad

- 1 cup of washed romaine or spinach in the bottom of a bowl
- In a frying pan melt 1 teaspoon of coconut oil and lightly sauté some onions, sweet peppers and garlic (spinach sautés nicely too)
- Scramble two free-range eggs in with the lightly cooked vegetables
- Place the cooked egg, onion, pepper and garlic mixture onto the bed of greens
- Top the salad with other produce like tomato and avocado

Note: Canning jars work great for traveling with layered salads or meals. And I can mass produce multiple servings at one time. I find that liquids are best on the bottom, the middle for produce, and nuts and grains layered at the top. Then if the preference is to eat the meal mixed up, simply shake the jar before removing the lid.

ME

What I also learned about combining foods is that a dish does not have to contain multiple ingredients. The meal itself might have just two separate items. For example, when my husband cooks flank steak, I prepare some asparagus to go with it. I learned that by chewing the meat with the vegetable together, the two items taste even better.

Here are some other examples of two-food combinations. I am not a huge fan of cucumbers. But if I slice them and place them on a whole-grain spelt cracker, it is a refreshing snack. Or carrots serve as a great alternative to bread, when wrapped with nitrate-free, organic lunchmeat.

By mixing foods that I don't recall ever trying together before, I learned to enjoy whole foods.

Don't Forget the Freezer

ME

I couldn't convince my family to eat the same meals I was eating. That left me preparing two meals every day—one for six people and one for just me. It was challenging to work all day, then come home and cook two meals that included whole grains, which took fifty minutes to cook. I found it to be a time saver to cook things like brown rice and meat in larger quantities on the weekends and freeze them in individual servings. In the mornings during the week, I thawed out the items that I planned on serving with fresh produce that evening.

Being from the Midwest my freezer also came in handy during the winter months. Over the summer, I purchased large quantities of organic, locally grown produce, such as blueberries, and froze them in small bags.

Note on whole grains: I really had to learn to read labels. Words like bleached and refined do not mean whole grains. They took the "whole" from it and served us the leftovers. Some examples of whole grains are

- Brown Rice
- Whole Oats
- Popcorn
- Muesli
- Wild Rice
- Amaranth
- Millet
- Quinoa
- Anything with the words Whole Wheat or Grain among the first ingredients

Take note of items not on this list: corn and flour tortillas, noodles, pita bread, white bread, and white rice. These choices typically do not include whole grains.

BC

I did not eat whole grains. I thought as long as I ate wheat bread instead of white that was sufficient.

TRI Here are two recipes. The first is a cilantro pesto that I use on whole grain pasta. Next is a recipe for some whole grain pancakes. The best part is that these pancakes can be frozen for future use. I just put them in my toaster to thaw in the morning.

Cilantro Pesto

- 1 clove garlic
- ½ cup almonds, cashews, or other nuts
- 1 cup fresh packed cilantro leaves (hold on to the bottom of the stem and pull toward the top to easily strip the leaves; I used to pluck each one individually)
- 2 tbsp lemon or lime juice
- 6 tbsp olive oil or flaxseed oil (I use 3tbsp of each)

Put the cilantro and the oil in the blender and mix this first and add the rest of the ingredients. Process until it is a lumpy paste. Add sea salt to taste. Unused portions freeze well.

Note: Cilantro and garlic are regarded as natural chelators. Chelators sweep away toxins and heavy metals.

Additional Note: I found an external use for flaxseed oil! It relieves the pain and relaxes my muscles from leg cramps. If I rub in some flax seed oil on the area that is tense, the muscles relax again within minutes.

Flax Cakes

- 2 tbsp virgin coconut oil
- 1 egg
- ¾ cup rice, almond, or hemp milk
- 3 tsp baking powder
- ½ tsp sea salt
- 1 cup whole grain organic spelt flour

Melt oil in pan. Place egg in mixing bowl. Beat. Then pour the melted, excess oil in the mixing bowl. Add all the rest of the ingredients except the flour and mix well with a fork. Add the flour and stir until lumps are mostly gone. Cook pancakes as normal, sprinkling ground flax seed on top before flipping.

Top the pancakes with pure maple syrup, raw honey, peanut butter, or sliced banana.

Stop the Runs

ME

My husband and I chuckle at family get-togethers where he looks at me and says, “What are you going to eat?” Everyone contributes their favorite side dish, which means there is a vast sea of yellow and white food to choose from. I realize that people want to bring a tasty, comforting dish to share. But I have not seen a gathering where families belly up to eat a heaping plate of green leafy vegetables.

Oftentimes, I have heard people discussing health issues and then they say, “Oh, you know cancer runs in the family.” Since being diagnosed, I have become more aware of health patterns in families. Some families suffer with chronic illnesses and some seem well. Living in a German community there is a good chance that many of us have Type A blood. So, then I wonder if Type A blood and the Midwestern diet are a lethal combination of potential health problems for some families. Remember 40 percent of the population has Type A blood and they are more prone to heart disease, cancer, and diabetes.

So, I am sitting right in the heart of this potential Type A blood mecca, and I hear doctors say that they do not understand why there are so many cancer cases in the Midwest. Could it be that we are in the heart of meat and potatoes land and Type As thrive as vegetarians? What a battle we may be facing without knowing the rules.

Another interesting consideration is that the problem isn’t exclusively type A blood, because most of the Japanese population have type A blood too. Yet, they have fewer cases of cancer and hardly any breast cancer. It is only when they move to the United States and eat the Standard American Diet that their cancer statistics migrate more toward U.S. levels. This screams out to me how correlated diet must be with chronic illness.

So, the question I keep asking is whether cancer runs in the family or if the risk is possibly more determined by our family’s eating habits? For example, let’s say I grew up eating hamburgers and cheesy potatoes for dinner. There is a greater chance I’d prepare the same type of meal for my family, as cooking habits are passed from generation to generation along with the increased risk of disease.

I am not picking on the Midwest or my family. What I am trying to illustrate is an empowering point. We may not have to succumb to the health patterns of our ancestors. Potentially, we could do the research for our children’s future and implement a plan for each person’s dietary needs. Then we could break the notion that “Cancer runs in our family.”

Consider this too. What do veterinarians change when our pets are sick? Their diet! The vet suggests that we purchase a certain kind of food to help the animal get better. Vets do it because there is a correlation between food and health. My wish is for more medical doctors to embrace and stress to their patients the importance of nutrition. Sometimes I wonder if our pets get better care than us.

From Carbonation to Hydration

ME

I wonder how I would feel if I washed the outside of my body with pop, iced coffee, and margaritas for a week. The idea of such an experiment seems pretty disgusting, but I did it every day to the inside of my body for years. I realize our society guides us to focus on the importance of the outer body, but in doing so, I disregarded the benefits of caring for myself from within.

When I changed my fluid intake exclusively to water, I noticed major changes in my physical health: less fatigue, sharper mind, more efficient digestion and elimination, fewer leg cramps, and clearer skin. But I also want to share a cancer-related testimony about the power of water. I made an awesome discovery when I realized drinking water took the discomfort away from my abdomen. Remember that I had multiple lesions on my liver. If I drank more water, I noticed I had less pain. It was empowering and uplifting to realize that I had some influence over this disease.

When I turned to water as my main source of hydration, I decided to drink either filtered water, reverse osmosis, or spring water. The filtered water was from my refrigerator, but there are many options available on the market for filtration. Please do not purchase a new fridge! There are products available as simple as filtrating pitchers.

My husband installed a reverse osmosis system under our kitchen sink. This form of water filtration can be found at most home improvement stores. Once it was installed, all we had to do was change the filters annually. Basically, I stay away from unfiltered tap water because most municipal sources add fluoride and chlorine, which I prefer to avoid because of the research I have done. Plus, some bottled waters are simply filled from these same municipal sources. That is why I typically choose spring water over purified water if I am away from home.

I discovered that we can protect ourselves from contaminants, not only from the water we drink, but also from the water we bathe in. Filters may also be installed in a shower head and are found at home improvement stores as well.

Note on bottled water: I store mine in a cool, dark place. I figure the sun, a plastic bottle, and my drinking water do not mix. Nor do I reuse containers that have the number one on the bottom, because bottles with a number one are intended to be used only once.

ME

After a while I got bored with just drinking water. I started adding green tea to my day because it has less caffeine than coffee or black tea. I find I sleep better without caffeine in my diet, and I do not want to jeopardize the quality of my sleep. There are many brands to choose from. One I especially like is Yogi. On the tab at the end of the string are uplifting phrases that rejuvenate me. I feel like I am opening a fortune cookie every time I have a cup.

TRI

People tell me all the time how great water is, but that they get headaches when they do not drink caffeine. I was the same way! Without caffeine in the morning, I suffered from crippling headaches by the afternoon. So, I bought caffeine pills at a drug store—the kind of pills that claim to keep us awake. Usually one pill has as much caffeine as one cup of coffee, which is around 200 mg for each dose. I took one in the morning for about a week. Then I broke one pill in half for the next week, and then progressed to a quarter of a pill, and so on. I was able to break the soft drink, coffee, and tea habit and still function. With the assistance of caffeine pills, I started drinking filtered water exclusively. And most importantly, I was sincerely grateful that I was not a slave to caffeine any longer.

BC

I drank pop, coffee, beer, and alcohol. If I drank water, it was minimal. And the water was not filtered. We stored our bottled water on a non-air-conditioned sun porch in direct sunlight. And my caffeine consumption was well over 400 mg per day.

Chapter Two
Incorporating Complementary and Alternative Therapies

The Power of Supplements

ME

I found it virtually impossible to rely on nutrition to sustain a high level of energy and manage the side effects from chemotherapy. It proved to be a continual balancing act to keep some of my blood test results within the normal range. From the time I was diagnosed there were nutrients that were low—for example, vitamin D. Then, during chemotherapy, my blood work revealed that magnesium and iron were below normal. I guess I could have maintained better results if I were even more militant in planning out every morsel of food that I ate, but who has time for that?

Being low in vitamin D seemed to be a commonality between me and other breast cancer survivors whom I had the privilege of meeting. Because of this, I feel strongly that patients and people with high risk for breast cancer should talk with their physicians about testing these levels. But don't just assume vitamin D is low because of the diagnosis; a simple blood test can detect the deficiency.

BC

Vitamin D was below normal. With the testing methodology used by my oncologist, the normal range was 32-100, and mine was at 25. Before this test, I did not take a vitamin D supplement, and I was hardly ever in the sun.

ME

Supplements were not only recommended to reverse deficiencies, they were also prescribed to prevent probable side effects from chemotherapy. Based on the input from my naturopath, chiropractor, and oncologist I also added supplements like:

- CoQ10 – to help my heart stay strong while I was on Herceptin
- Vitamin B – for the neuropathy (numbness) in my toes
- Astragulus – for general immune system support

- Melatonin – as a sleep aid. I took 20 mg per night.

There were other supplements integrated into my care too, but I share this partial list just as a reminder that professionals recommend natural food supplements that are tailored to each person's special needs and treatment plan. I was incredibly thankful I nurtured my body with the use of supplements and not more drugs.

Listed above are the core supplements that helped me during chemotherapy, but I have to tell a short story about one of them in particular, melatonin. After I was diagnosed with cancer, my naturopath recommended that I take melatonin every day before bedtime. I took it regularly for a while, but then I got lazy and began to skip it more often than not. When I admitted to my naturopath that I had neglected to take the sleep aid, he said that if he were stranded on a desert island with cancer and could only take one supplement with him, it would be melatonin. After that, I was a little more motivated to fit it back into my late evening routine.

RE I read in *The New Bible Cure for Cancer*, by Don Colbert, MD, "Melatonin has been shown to improve immune system function, help individuals cope with stress, and diminish certain aspects of aging, as well as help fight fibrocystic breast diseases and breast and colon cancers. It also demonstrates protection against the toxic side effects of chemotherapy and radiation therapy and improves healing after cancer surgery."

TRI At times the number of supplements got excessive, and consequently, they made me feel mildly nauseated. This was most noticeable when I took them on an empty stomach or during the first few days after chemotherapy. I asked my chiropractor if I could grind the tablets up in a blender and drink them with liquid. He gave me the great idea of putting the vitamins through a coffee grinder first and then adding the vitamin powder to the blender with fresh squeezed juice. I did as he suggested. For the capsules I cut the tip open with scissors and poured the contents directly into the blender with the ground tablets and the juice. I felt as if my body was utilizing the blended nutrients more efficiently. I seemed to have more energy and minimal nausea. Plus, I was free from swallowing all those capsule casings. That alone must provide some kind of health benefit!

I have to admit this vitamin–infused, blended juice drink was challenging to the palate, but it only lasted a few seconds besides being easier for me than digesting a bunch of caplets. I did not invest in a very expensive grinder. Because vitamin tablets are not as dense as coffee beans, an inexpensive grinder worked fine.

ME I also learned it is not always best to take supplements. I asked my chiropractor about selenium because I had seen it mentioned in a lot of cancer prevention/fighting books. He said not to take a supplement, but rather, eat a couple Brazil nuts every day. Two Brazil nuts have 140-180 micrograms of selenium. It is suggested to have 200 mcg per day. Sometimes supplements are not the preferred option, even by chiropractors. Sometimes the ideal solution is found in food.

Note on Brazil nuts: I do not eat them every day because Brazil nuts are not compatible with Type A blood (visit Dr. D'Adamo's website, www.dadamo.com, for more information about the blood-type diet). But because they are a good cancer fighter, I eat them a couple times a week.

A year after treatment stopped, I needed some adrenal gland support. I felt my energy slipping and my sleep quality was relatively poor. I switched to Celtic sea salt, and my energy bounced right back. No drugs and no vitamins, and I felt better within days. Celtic sea salt is good for electrolyte support, naturally lower in sodium, and full of minerals and trace elements.

BC The only salt in my diet was from processed foods. I thought salt was bad for my health. I rarely used a salt shaker. I did not realize that salt could be good for me, and that there were benefits of using sea salt over traditional options.

I rarely ate Brazil nuts unless someone served a dish of mixed nuts at a party.

Note: To find a naturopath who specializes in cancer, visit the websites of the Oncology Association of Naturopathic Physicians (www.oncanp.org) or the American Association of Naturopathic Physicians (www.naturopathic.org).

All in One

ME

My chiropractor provided the convenience of multiple kinds of treatments that complemented my care. I felt like I was at the spa not only for the outside of my body, but for the inside. I had researched the cancer fighting properties of certain supplements. But I turned to him for guidance on which ones to take, and I was grateful for his opinions and expertise. The other reason I chose to drive 60 minutes to meet with him was his use of some unique techniques to determine the needs of his patients.

The human body has the ability to provide guidance for healing and balance. My chiropractor uses Contact Reflex Analysis (CRA), sometimes called muscle testing, to reveal the root of problems that modern medicine may miss. CRA uncovers information within the body through its own electrical signals. When the system is in balance, CRA will not find anything. However, when a certain joint, organ, or bone is not working properly, or is misaligned, the body sends a signal to that area. This is what CRA detects, and practitioners then do what they can to bring the problem area back in balance. These interventions may include chiropractic adjustments, supplementation, acupuncture, and more.

I rediscovered the diagnostic power of CRA when I was finished with chemotherapy and started taking Tamoxifen, a prescription drug taken daily to lower estrogen levels. The test revealed that my liver needed help processing the drug. Coincidentally, I attended a symposium at the University of Illinois a couple months later. This panel of researchers found that some patients do not benefit from Tamoxifen because the liver does not break down the drug properly. But because of my chiropractor's work, this issue had already been addressed and fixed by prescribing a supplement to enhance my liver function. If we had not discovered my system's ineffectiveness in processing this drug, the outcome may have been similar to the neutral effect of taking a placebo.

His testing also included the use of a Zyto machine. Like muscle testing, this machine does not diagnose disease, but rather it monitors stressors in the body by means of a process called "biosurvey." This biosurvey is done by cradling the hand on a metal reader, which looks like the outline of a glove. In a matter of minutes, the body communicates with the computer and provides the doctor with valuable information, including which supplements and alternative therapies to incorporate into the patient's care. This system also generates a report that is reviewed at the office and sent to the patient by email. It was helpful for me to look back on these reports from time to time and monitor trends. Another valuable feature of a Zyto scan is that it reads food intolerances. Sometimes food choices add systemic stress.

Not only did my chiropractor assist me with supplementation throughout cancer treatment, but when needed, he adjusted my spine. His examination would alert him when a subluxation (misalignment) was present. His manipulation of the spine removed the interference from within my nervous system. I like to think of his work this way: If a garden hose is pinched, the water does not arrive at its destination as intended. The spinal cord is the same way. When misalignments happen, organs do not function at their full potential, and health deteriorates.

Occasionally, he also used acupuncture during my visits to balance the energy within my body. It was extremely relaxing. Frequently when the session was over, he had to wake me up.

The beauty of the chiropractors' work is that they acknowledge they are not healers, but that they help facilitate the healing process. They say their job is to remove the interference and allow us to function at a higher and more efficient level. They stand in awe of the power of the nervous system and witness the transformation of their clients.

My point in sharing all this is to show that chiropractors have many different tools to assist us. I have friends whom I have taken to the chiropractor and he never adjusts them or sticks needles in them. The visit is customized to their preferences, because the patient is in charge! After seeing compelling results for myself, I hold an intense belief about the immeasurable benefits of having a chiropractor on my team. Don't let the fear of their cracking your neck keep you away.

The costs vary throughout the country for these types of treatments. In the heart of Illinois, I usually pay forty to one hundred dollars for these services. One thing I do know is chiropractors do not do this for the money. If they did, they could certainly charge a lot more! I have introduced friends to alternative therapies, and for most it is a hard transition. Oftentimes, the deal breaker is that the services are not typically covered by insurance. But I am perplexed as I look at our society and witness the massive amounts of attention placed on outward appearances. We think nothing of spending money for weight loss, fashion items, and eating out at fancy restaurants, but won't spend the same amount to take care of the inside of our bodies. It is almost as if our attitude is that if we do not see it, it doesn't exist or require attention.

Note: If you are still questioning the healing power of the body, think of the last time there was a small cut on your hand. Did the bandage heal you, or did your body? Everything we do has the potential to facilitate a different level of wellness. Sometimes it needs the helping hand of a holistic professional.

I Kept Moving

ME

I chose walking as my form of exercise. I could do it anytime and anywhere. I did not have to invest in a gym membership or be at a fitness class three times a week. I appreciated the flexibility that walking offered, because I already had plenty of structure. Days were filled with work, meetings, church activities, kid's games, volleyball matches, and now, coping with cancer. I did not need one more scheduled activity to add to my calendar.

There were times I did not walk very far. Surgery and my first chemotherapy treatment proved to be difficult for me, and there were days when all I could do was walk up and down the hallway of our home. The next day I felt a little better and walked into the living room and back multiple times with rests in between. After a couple more days I added some steps. And walked up and down our driveway, and then to the corner. I kept pushing myself a little farther every day. A year and eight days after diagnosis I walked in my first half marathon completing 13.1 miles in less than four hours. And it all started by walking a just few feet in our hallway.

I even kept moving during most of my infusions of chemotherapy. I just rolled the IV cart beside me and strolled through the hallways of the clinic. I did so much walking the nurses nicknamed me "The Walker." It made the time go by. I wonder if it was beneficial during infusion because the chemotherapy flowed through a moving body better than if I were sedentary. I don't have any proof of it, but it makes me ponder on the possibility. Universities are doing studies on walking and breast cancer reoccurrence. So, is it possible that walking during chemotherapy could produce more preferable outcomes too?

During the winter of 2011, I trained at the mall for the half marathon. I appreciated that this environment was warm, dry, and safe and that the building opens three hours early to accommodate walkers. The distance for one lap around the entire mall was almost one mile. While I was training, I placed coins in my pocket for the number of miles I wanted to accomplish. If I planned for a five-mile walk, I started with five pennies in my pocket. Every time I passed by the water fountain in the food court I pulled a penny out of my pocket, made a wish, and dropped it in the fountain. When the pennies were gone, I was done. This allowed me more spiritual time rather than keeping track of how many laps I still needed to accomplish.

While writing this book, I took my computer tablet with me to the mall in a backpack or handbag. Then I could jot down notes whenever I needed a break. Since there were limited distractions, the environment was conducive to reflection and creativity. And it was a great way to multitask.

Walking also gave me an opportunity to detoxify. My dad and I planned excursions to Turkey Run State Park in Indiana. A couple days before my scheduled treatments we would hike in the afternoon. He'd say, "It's time to blow out the old and get ready for the new." With this one activity I worked my body, sweated out toxins, and spent some quality time with my dad in a beautiful state park.

Yet another benefit of walking was relief from achy legs. In November of 2010, while I was on both Herceptin and Tamoxifen, I experienced a dull, constant ache from the waist down. This feeling was more intense the longer I sat. But I found movement provided a break from the discomfort. Initially it was difficult to convince myself to start moving when the entire lower half of my body was uncomfortable, but I quickly learned that it subsided while I was in motion. Sitting in a meeting or a conference was close to unbearable. When I attended our children's ball games and sat in the bleachers, I walked the halls of the school during halftime. I was certainly surprised to find the remedy came from doing the opposite of what I expected or felt like doing.

I remember when, as a kid, I was sick for a day and had to stay in bed. I felt weak the next day from lying around. Chemotherapy was similar. There were times to rest, but there was also a time to move.

What I read in the Bible reminded me that people walked everywhere, sometimes for weeks and years. It reinforced the idea that we were not designed to sit in recliners or lie around in bed. Our bodies are vehicles made by our creator for motion and activity. Cancer does not change that. We may have to adapt, but we do not have to do without.

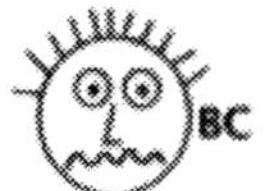

I pushed myself pretty hard with my workouts. I felt walking was a waste of time.

WAY Once, I received a timely gift—a stray dog we named Sadie. She was a well-trained and compassionate dog that showed up at our farm about the same time I was getting bored walking the mall. It was spring time and I yearned to walk outside, but the reality of walking the same country road over and over again left me hard-pressed to stay motivated. Then Sadie arrived. It was as if she was sent to me by God, and the timing was impeccable.

Believed to be a red heeler, which is bred for herding, and terrier mix, she was a great companion that required minimal discipline or a leash. She was free to hop through the fields, and she kept me entertained during our evening strolls together. She showered me with love and the motivation to keep moving. I was not looking for a dog; she found me.

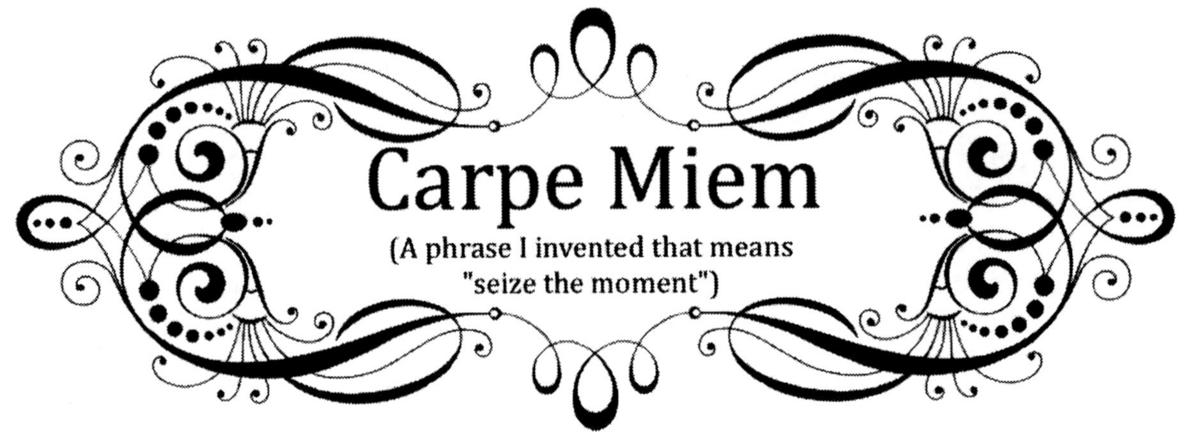

Carpe Miem

(A phrase I invented that means "seize the moment")

The moment I learned of my diagnosis my mind raced *way* too far in the future. To say my life's plan was shattered was an understatement. My father still reminds me of when I gave him my financial statement within minutes of being diagnosed with Stage IV cancer. He looked at me like I was acting ridiculous. But I was in panic mode, and I felt that I had to get all my affairs in order. Once I got past that initial shock and grasped that I was not going to die in days, I searched all of humanity for solutions only to find out that no one but God really knew the answers to the big questions. When I realized that looking into the future and questioning the past was a waste of time, I decided to change my mantra to "Today is beautiful," with a big period. I didn't go much past that. At night I sincerely and gratefully prayed for the gifts I received that day. Very rarely did I pray about what I wished for in the future, but rather I expressed my appreciation for the aspects of the day that guided me toward God's will.

My life became more easygoing, when I decided to live in the moment. I woke up in the morning and thought about the opportunities that were in store for me. What could I offer the world today? I constantly reminded myself that my intentions should not be tainted with the worry that I may not be here six months, because today was here! It proved to be a difficult transition to make. But once I arrived at the other side, I felt peaceful. I focused on being grateful for today's progress. If people asked how I was doing, I would answer "Today is beautiful!" The best part is that I found this simple response steered acquaintances away from asking questions about the future or sharing stories about how their family members succumbed to a gruesome death from the disease. It truly helped me get through the workweek with a more positive spirit.

I attended a Breast Cancer Recovery retreat in the Wisconsin Dells a couple years after I was diagnosed. During this time I realized that even though I may not be cured, I could achieve a higher level of serenity by being mindful, which simply means remaining attentive and aware. Instead of getting caught up in my own mind, I learned to live in harmony with, and exist in, each moment.

Within minutes of gathering at the retreat, the session leader asked us what we planned to accomplish during our four days together. Without hesitation I answered, "I want to learn how to take a breath." I had been on this fight-or-flight roller coaster ride for months; it was time to get off. A year into remission, I needed to live again. And I knew God wanted this second chance to be a special experience for me, a life richer than I had ever imagined. Why go through all this to return to where I came from? In order to accomplish my mission I knew I had to start with learning how to stop my mind from racing—or looping, as some called it. So, that was my objective: for the next 72 hours—practice living in the moment.

I awoke the next morning eager to infuse "carpe miem," my phrase for living in the moment, into my day. I grabbed my muffin and tea, switched on the fireplace and grabbed a floor pillow. I sat in front of the hearth taking in the moment. Trying, with great difficulty, to watch the flames dance and savor every flavor in the food I was eating, the five minutes of mindfulness seemed like an eternity. But I figured just like when I started walking up and down our hallway for exercise, learning to live in the moment required baby steps too.

As uncomfortable as my first attempt was, I decided to keep trying. I opened my window shade to view the nature that surrounded the spa. In the distance along the edge of the nearby woods, I saw the back half of a deer behind a tree. Normally I would notice it and say, "That's neat," and go on with my business. But reminding myself—training myself—to stay in this moment, I was blessed to see a second deer join the first. Carpe Miem was working! And eventually, to my surprise, a third deer showed up.

Witnessing the third deer immediately filled my heart with joy when I remembered that the number three is a symbol of healing and wholeness. I believe the number three points to the fullness of God and life. Taking a moment to notice that third deer reassured me that I was on the right track, and that the healing of my soul was closely related to living in the moment.

I was on a role, so rather than meeting with other attendees for breakfast, I decided to walk the grounds of the resort. It was on the cusp of our first full day together. So, in my old fashioned routine, I allowed questions to race through my head like, "I wonder what we are going to talk about?" "I wonder if I will connect with another survivor?" "I wonder if my story will inspire others?" In my head I yelled out a huge, SSSSTTTTOOOPPPPPP!!!! Because when I gave into to those powerful voices, precious moments were lost forever. As soon as I snapped out of the unpleasant existence that originated from my racing mind, a pine needle dropped out of the tree and lodged into the mastectomy side of my asymmetrical cleavage. Since I spent the summers in Maine surrounded by millions of pine needles, I considered this simple pine needle to be a sign from above—a physical reminder that there is healing that comes from living in the moment. During the rest of my walk, I noticed birds, the wind whistling through the trees, and the fresh smells of nature, not my thoughts about the future.

The night before our departure I was emotionally saturated from the events of the retreat. I was eager to practice more mindfulness. So, I headed to town by car to explore a path that led me to a river. I could see I was making progress, but continually had to remind myself to pay attention to nature's show. I took pictures of flowers and the scenery by the river. I decided a great way to document my carpe miem baby steps was to capture moments with photos. I touched some bark on a tree. It occurred to me that I had not even touched a tree in years. So, I took a photo of this rare event.

As I closed my computer tablet another photo snapped. Being an orderly person, there was no way I could allow a picture of nothing to remain in the memory. During the process of attempting to delete this photo, I noticed the time in the corner was 3:33.

I decided to keep that photo after all.

Not Only In but On

ME

Not only do I watch what I put *in* my body, but I am selective of the products I put *on* my body. I was shocked to learn how efficiently our skin absorbs hygiene and beauty products when I had a scan done at my chiropractor's office to test for food allergies. Interestingly enough, spearmint came up as a food to avoid. It was nothing I ever consumed, but I had been using it on my skin in the form of natural soap. I thought if spearmint came up positive for allergies, what other products with man-made additives did my system have trouble processing over the years? This test reinforced that I not only needed to read labels to nurture my body from the inside out but also from the outside in.

After I transformed my diet, I started switching out my toiletries to options with natural ingredients. I found alternatives for toothpaste, deodorant, soap, shampoo, hair gel, make-up, and sunscreen. I am not suggesting these products are perfect. But they are better than what I had been using in the past, and after weeks of trial and error these are the brands I prefer:

- **Toothpaste –** Nature's Gate, Wintergreen Gel, found at health food stores.
  Note: Switching to a non-fluoride option did not cause the cavities I might have feared.
- **Deodorant –** Tom's roll-on, citrus zest, found in health and drug stores.
  Note: Since I migrated to a plant-based diet, I can almost get away without deodorant. It is as if I exude cleanliness from the inside out.
- **Soap/Hair Care –** There are many natural products to choose from for bar soap, liquid soap and shampoo, but I have enjoyed using Dr. Bronner's soaps. My hair has remained short. So, I use the liquid version from head to toe. It is all natural and a little goes a long way, and a large bottle lasts months. Dr. Bronner's is easiest to find in health food stores. Though it comes in many scents, our favorite is almond.
- **Hair Gel –** Flaxseed Hi Shine by Jason can be found at Whole Foods. It holds my short hair in place for hours.
- **Make up –** I have gravitated to options found at the health food stores and companies like Arbonne, which is a multi-level marketing company that specializes in more natural products.
- **Sunscreen –** With Arbonne's damage control, water-resistant, SPF 30, I can be in the sun longer than with traditional products, and I do not have to apply a lot of the product to my skin.

- **Lubricant –** Hormone therapy forced me to make some adjustments regarding intimacy. I found a natural and friendly alternative in pure vitamin E oil, which I purchase at drug and health stores.

Note: I avoid beauty products with parabens. Parabens are used to inhibit the growth of bacteria, mold and yeast, but are far from natural. The products that used to be in my bathroom cabinets included ingredients like methylparaben, propylparaben, butylparaben, and ethylparaben, which I now refrain from using.

Relief and Detox from Massage and Wraps

ME

Massage helped relieve the nausea and body aches that resulted from chemotherapy. I suffered from leg aches that were similar to the growing pains of when I was a child—the dull ache that did not go away no matter what I tried. Fortunately, I found relief by having a massage about five to six days after each of my treatments. I did not schedule it any sooner because I didn't want to flush the chemotherapy from my body prematurely. After having a session and consuming lots of water, most of the side effects subsided. Since chemotherapy ended, I still have a massage once a month for relaxation and detoxifying.

Based on my diagnosis, the oncologist advised against deep tissue massage. She did not believe that would be good for me, since the cancer was throughout my body and there was an increased risk of spreading the disease further. Even after I went into remission, I continued to refrain from deep tissue work.

My massage therapist is also trained in the therapeutic uses of body wraps. She applies oils with herbal compounds to extract toxins through the skin. After slathering me up, she literally wraps me in plastic, and lets the mixture work for about twenty to thirty minutes.

I experienced my first body wrap in the spring of 2011, a couple of months after I finished my first complete round of chemotherapy. I remember being extremely cold during this treatment. When she removed the plastic the room smelled like chemotherapy, even though it had been a while since my last infusion. I tried a wrap again about a year later. This time I did not feel nearly as cold, and she reassured me the odor was similar to that of normal, smelly people toxins.

Note: Body wraps may not be beneficial if you suffer from claustrophobia. I was wrapped up pretty tightly.

BC

I had enjoyed massage on rare occasions before diagnosis, but I did not feel it was worth the money, and I certainly did not make the time for myself.

Our Kids Know Better

ME

Our kids love to go barefoot in the summer. It used to frustrate me, because being unused to farm life, I thought that it was dirty, and I was afraid they were going to absorb some kind of creeping crud through their feet. I had to pick my battles though. Come to find out, they were right! Instinctually, children know what their bodies need to thrive without being taught. They recognize that they benefit from the earth's energy, even though we adults just call it messy.

I learned a valuable lesson through the actions of our children. Kids do not let the world dictate what is right. Sometimes they simply do what feels right. It reminds me of the movie *Pretty Woman*, when Julia Roberts had to coerce Richard Gere to take his shoes off in the park and feel the grass. How did Americans get so disconnected from the earth?

Earthing is a recent discovery and remedy for this disconnection, and is based on the study of ancient lifestyles. Back in biblical times, man walked barefoot and slept on the earth. We were in constant contact with the ground then, but nowadays we hardly touch it. We sleep in homes, sometimes multiple stories high, and walk in shoes that insulate us from the earth's surface. Not only are we disconnected from the protection of the earth's energy, but we work in buildings with equipment that emit electromagnetic energy. This energy could be neutralized if we were in contact with the ground. But if we have an office job, that could be next to impossible without the help of Earthing products.

Clinton Ober discovered the benefits of being connected to the earth and developed products to help us establish that connection. There are many testimonials from people who were able to reverse symptoms of disorders such as MS, fibromyalgia, arthritis, autism, lupus, jet lag, poor circulation, sciatica, sleep apnea, arrhythmias, and stress by simply connecting to earth's energy again.

Earthing, the book by Clinton Ober, taught me that Earthing is simply a neutralizing of positive and negative energy. The free radicals in our body are positively charged and the earth is negatively charged. When we come in contact with the ground, this effect is neutralized, and the body functions more efficiently.

This book was one of my favorites. But there is also information on www.earthing.com or at www.earthinginstitute.net about this theory. These sites also sell grounding products that I have used in the comfort of my home, since I am not a big fan of outdoor living. My husband and I have slept on sheets connected to the earth for months. I sleep better and my mind does not race as much when I wake up in the middle of the night. These sheets are pricey but so convenient. The pads come in handy when I stay in hotels for a long period of time. I use the mouse pad while I work at the credit union and the bands around my ankle while I write. These are all great products with unique uses, but I really like the sheets. Because we sleep grounded, I am connected at least one third of the day.

The websites also market outlet testers to ensure that your outlet is truly grounded. The Earthing products connect to a wire plugged into the ground of your electrical socket. The ground is the round hole in the three-hole outlet. There is no electrical current in this opening, because it provides a connection to the earth that is independent of the current-carrying path. We found the outlet tester to be helpful for confirmation that our outlets were grounded. If they were not, the customer can purchase another product sold by these websites, which provide a ground through a cord with a metal rod that is strung through a nearby window and stuck in the dirt outside.

If I lived in a warmer climate, I might have accomplished better results by actually touching the ground. Walking barefoot, sitting on the ground to meditate, or swimming in the ocean are great way to connect with the healing properties of the earth. Since I did not live in a warm climate, I purchased Earthing products for the winter months. If I didn't have those products, I could have placed my bare feet on the unpainted, slightly damp cement floor of our basement.

Notes on Earthing and Medications: There are precautions in the book for people taking thyroid medicine or Coumadin, which is a blood thinner. They suggest that your doctor should know about your plans to start Earthing. Ober's research revealed some people can drop these medications or lessen the dosage, but the adjustments must be done with the advice of your doctor.

An Additional Safety Note: Earthing products should be *unplugged during thunderstorms*.

Sleep

ME

I have valued sleep quality and quantity since my diagnosis. I credit many factors for improving my sleep. First, I try to go to sleep and wake up around the same time every day. I feel it decreases systemic stress if my body knows what to expect. Secondly, I reflected on the times of my life that I rested the best. I thought it was because of the varying levels of stress in my life, but now I believe it could have been related to positioning. And finally, I curbed my habit of eating and snacking before bedtime to improve sleep quality.

I also invested in a new bed. I ordered one through my chiropractor that resembles the highly advertised brand that is made of foam. Ours is similar, but it is made from natural materials including organic cotton. Because of government regulations, beds are manufactured with fire resistant chemicals. Thankfully, this brand does not have those added chemicals. I now sleep wonderfully and do not wake up every time my husband moves. If it fixed his snoring, it would be a super bed!

After buying the new bed, I was sleeping well, but I still yearned for a better quality sleep. My prayers were answered when it was suggested to me that the direction I face while sleeping could have a strong effect upon my wellbeing.

I reflected on the direction of my slumber over the years. I recalled the best results were when I slept north, which was how I slept as a teenager. I slept facing east before our wedding day. I thought I had trouble sleeping during this time because of all the planning for the wedding. We changed our bed to the south a couple months later, and I slept better. But at the time, I thought it was because the wedding was over, and I was moved in. Then we rotated to the north to test my theory, and I slept even better.

One day my husband and I decided to change our room so that our heads were facing east again. Whoa, was that a wrong choice! I slept horribly again. We switched the bed back to the north, and I slept like a baby. Based on my own experience the only direction I avoid, even in a hotel, is west. The times I have slept in this way have been some of the darkest moments in my life. If the headboard is facing west, I flip around and sleep with my head toward the footboard. To remember, I alliterate "west is worst."

The hardest change I made to improve my sleep was to refrain from nighttime snacking. But I made the change because I now know that if I eat before resting for the night, more energy is expended on digesting food rather than healing and repairing my body from the events of the day. Plus, I do not sleep as well on a full stomach.

This was a hard habit to break until I found chamomile tea. I can curb my snacking late at night with a cup before bedtime. The chamomile flower is a natural relaxant. The hot tea calms me and helps extinguish those late night cravings.

Note: If you are allergic to ragweed, there may be side effects from the tea.

BC Late at night I snacked on ice cream, dessert, or an apple with peanut butter. I perceived food as a reward for a challenging day. And the more difficult the day, the less nutritional my food choices were. I considered it a good night's sleep when I woke up in the middle of the night and fell back asleep within two hours. But I did not notice the relationship between bad habits like eating late and being hyped up on caffeine and my sleep quality. I rarely fell asleep before 10 or 11 o'clock.

Bio Cranial Therapy

RE Bio Cranial Therapy, as I understand it, is based on correcting what my practitioner refers to as the Master System. He explained to me that even though science tells us these plates fuse as we age, experts in cranial therapy believe that the bones in the skull still move. So let's assume these plates are able to move slightly. But if they are restricted and not allowed to flow freely, it may cause problems for many of the systems of the body. Cranial therapy relieves this limited mobility.

ME The procedure took five to ten minutes. The therapy was done in two steps, once on the left side of the upper part of my neck and again on the right. My neck was manipulated, but unlike a chiropractic adjustment, it was more like intense stretching. I had a moment to feel the difference in my body after he finished the first side, and from my head to my toes that entire side felt peaceful, tranquil and at rest. The right side, on the other hand, was still very busy—like static on TV. After the right side was adjusted, I felt light—physically and mentally. I went home and did not think too much about the changes, but I enjoyed my relaxed state all evening.

In the middle of the night I got up, like I normally do, to go to the bathroom. Usually, I gingerly get out of bed because of my years of volleyball—or so I assumed that was the issue. But that night I popped right out of bed. By correcting the Master System, my entire body readjusted to being more aligned *all the way down to my knees.*

My head has been much clearer since the procedure. The biggest change I noticed, though, was that I sing songs in my head more than before. In the past, my thoughts have been filled with meaningless garbage like, "What about this?" and "What about that?" The treatment helped me live more in the moment.

I may not require the therapy again, because my imbalance may have been created at birth. It is amazing to think that Cranial Therapy may have corrected something I have lived with my entire life, and in just one session.

Reike, Wow! What a Trip

ME

A close family friend scheduled an appointment for me to have a Reike treatment. Reike is basically rebalancing energy. The Reike master lived three hours away and knew nothing about me ahead of time. Before she began, she asked, "Do you want me to tell you what I feel as I go along, or do you prefer silence?" Of course, I was curious, so I told her I wanted to learn as much as I could. As soon as the session began, she went directly to my right leg. She said it felt as if there was static or mini lightning bolts radiating from my right knee. I had fallen one week earlier from roller skating because my bearings locked up.

Next she said it felt like there was a speed bump by my liver. And that is where some of the tumors were. She also said that she believed there was a connection between my liver and my ears. Ironically, before the cancer diagnosis, I had suffered from chronic skin irritation in my ear, which had ended up going away with proper diet. I was amazed she found it with Reike, since I had been asymptomatic for a year.

Then while over the area of the mastectomy, and yes, she was on the correct side, she compared the energy to something gushing out of me. I told her that is where my surgery was for breast cancer. She responded, "Ok, we will just shut that back up." She proceeded to make motions as if she was containing the energy that I had been leaking around the left side of my chest since the surgery and pushing it back in to regain control.

She found one more specific area that needed attention. She said that there was something strange toward the front of my brain. Not sure what that meant, but I did suffer from seizures as a child.

That was all she said. It was very spiritual and inexplicably astounding, especially since she knew nothing about my health issues.

When I went for the second treatment, almost a year later, I had been in remission for 9 months. This time, she said my body was quiet. For me this corroborated the scan results from days earlier, which revealed that there was no evidence of disease.

Life After Chemo

ME

For me, as a cancer survivor, the journey was not a sprint but a marathon. I knew if I made changes and reverted back to my old habits, my life could be in jeopardy again. My new lifestyle was about rebirth. The cancer was not just the tumor in my breast, but rather a systemic warning that I had been in desperate need of an overhaul. At the very least I needed to continue with the changes I had made.

I still do the following items on the following schedule as maintenance. It is not a chore. It is part of being the person I value caring for—the renewed me.

- **Chiropractic –** when needed, but at least once a month
- **Acupuncture –** occasionally, but not as often as chiropractic adjustments
- **Massage –** monthly, usually ninety-minute sessions
- **Body Wraps –** every six to twelve months
- **Earthing –** daily
- **Reike –** every six to twenty-four months
- **Cranial Therapy –** twice in the last few years
- **Walking –** two miles, three to five times per week
- **Sleep –** in bed by nine and asleep by ten, wake on my own at seven
- **Nutrition –** still eat the same diet, and I rarely "treat" myself

I understand all this may seem like a huge expense, but I do not think of it that way. Money was the least of my worries. I wanted to achieve wellness without cost as a deciding factor. Since I was Stage IV, maybe it was easier for me to part with the money? Perhaps. I prefer to think I migrated toward a healthier balance of saving for the future and enjoying the resources that God gave me. I now live more for today, and do not hoard money for tomorrow. The lesson I learned was that when I take the time to take care of myself, I have the energy to give more and love more.

Part Two

Redefine, Reinvent, and Recreate, Despite Unfavorable Odds

When I was first diagnosed, my spirit was dampened by the urge to figure out why this happened to me. But then I realized that I was wasting time seeking the answers to a question that could not be answered. Instead, I decided that the quality of my life depended on how I coped and adapted. This lesson was unveiled within minutes of being diagnosed. The following story depicts that moment, and it was as if God was saying, "I got you! Trust in me."

His Name was Chet

I vividly remember the day I was diagnosed. I was at work when I received the phone call. As soon as I heard the phrase "Your test came back positive," it instantly demolished my dreams as a newlywed. When I retell the story of that exact moment with other survivors, I am reminded of the portrayal of the teacher from Charlie Brown, "You have blah, blah carcinoma in your blah, blah." Once I heard the word positive, my mind started racing. I completely stopped listening. All I heard was that one key word, and I proceeded to draw my own conclusions about the rocky and uncertain path that lay before me. I freaked out!

I hung up the phone and attempted to gather my composure and face the world for the first time with cancer. I looked at our vice president and simply said, "I've got it."

He responded, "Well, we have a member here for a loan and another member who needs to open an account." He gave me two choices, neither of which I wanted to hear, because I would have preferred running out of the office screaming like my hair was on fire. But after 25 years of serving others, I gathered my composure and joined the couple wanting to open a new account.

They were a young couple, recently married and new to town. I collected the pertinent information on the primary member. Then I turned to the joint owner. He handed me his driver's license. His name was Chet. My grandfather's name was Chet. In all my years of managing thousands of accounts I had never seen that name on any of them.

My grandfather greatly influenced my life. He took me to his campsite in Maine near Lake Sebago for weeks at a time, just him and me. I thought every grandchild got to spend that much time with their grandfathers. I realized years later how fortunate I was to have his loving influence in my life.

When I saw the name Chet on this member's ID, it immediately brought me back to the feelings I had over thirty years ago. I felt guidance, safety, and love. Here was my first gift from God within seconds of receiving a cancer diagnosis. In an instant, He let me know that I was loved and in His hands as I was years earlier by my grandfather. My first lesson taught me not to freak out but to trust.

If I had run out of the credit union crying and losing my mind, I would have missed this beautiful gift. So, from that point on I decided to live the best life I could and live in harmony with cancer rather than letting cancer control me. And most importantly I recognized the gifts that come when I listen and trust in Him.

Chapter Three
Rebuilding Spirit From Within

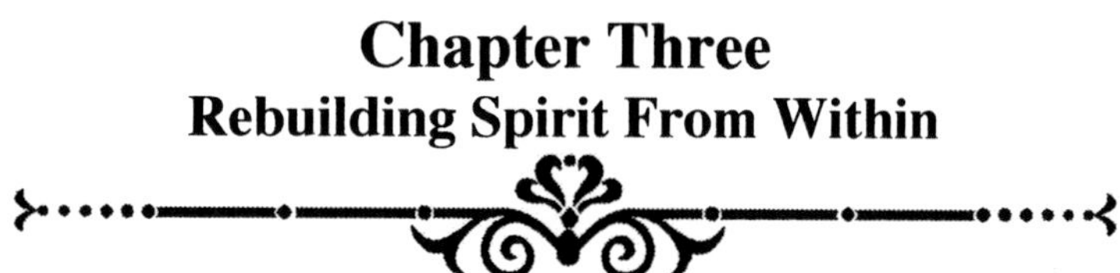

Who Wants to Hang Out With a Grump?

ME

I chose to accept, enjoy, and be more enthusiastic about life. The only other option was depression, which encouraged others to be miserable with me. When I was first diagnosed, I quickly learned that loved ones follow my lead. For instance:

- If I act like a victim, the world labels me as one.
- If I am negative, my family exudes similar energy.
- If I display sadness, my friends cry with me.

Family and friends patterned themselves after my emotional style because they loved me and wanted to be supportive. So, I started to shape my attitude to mirror the energy that I want those around me to exhibit. I found that if I oozed with hope and promise, my loved ones emulated similar emotions. And we were all more hopeful.

Besides, "Who wants to hang out with a grump?" I knew if the roles were reversed, I would be hard-pressed to spend a great amount of time with someone who was always down. If I detoured down the road of despair, that question reminded me of the big picture.

Because the answer is...no one.

Releasing Stress and Duress

BC Life before diagnosis was stressful, as it is for many. To illustrate where I came from, I share an account of a typical day.

The months preceding diagnosis were more demanding of my time than normal, as I tried to adjust to many life-changing events. I was the president of a credit union, which was not new, but we experienced turnover recently in some key positions. During this time we fully remodeled the main office after 25 years. It needed it. I was engaged and had invited close to four hundred guests for a weekend wedding extravaganza, which involved a rehearsal dinner, a dessert reception at church, a small gathering at a local restaurant, and a huge party at our home the next day. Before the nuptials I sold the home of my dreams, transferred all my belongings to storage, and moved in with a friend. Then I got married and I literally transitioned to my new life with my husband and his three children overnight.

Eating excessively provided comfort and was my main coping mechanism. My own food pyramid, which in actuality resembled a rectangle, was molded by the fast-food that I ate in the car. Most mornings I had iced coffee and a plain bagel with egg. During my lunch hour I traveled to the gym for weightlifting. On the way back I stopped at a sub shop and ordered a foot-long sandwich. I ate half of it in the car while I drove back to work and ate the other half that evening on the way to one of our children's ball games. Yes, there were many days that all of my meals were consumed in the car. The food I ate lacked nutrition, none of it was alive, and it offered no variety. I was a creature of habit, and my diet matched my lifestyle.

On the rare occasion that I ate at home, it was typically right before bedtime. I am embarrassed to say there were many nights I found temporary relief by using dessert as an unsuitable reward for a stressful day.

I rarely drank water. My fluids consisted of caffeinated coffee and soda.

I slept horribly. The worry over all the unprecedented factors in my life had overwhelmed me, to the point that one night, I awoke to find my hands clenched so tightly that I had fingernail marks in my palms.

I was a physical and emotional worn-out mess!

ME I've met many cancer survivors who endured major stressors before the onset of illness, but few grasped the possible correlation. It seemed as if many of those survivors had experienced life changes such as family issues, financial problems, divorce, loss of job, death in the family etc., usually stressors beyond their control. Life changes are common for everyone, but some manage it better than others. I was not one of them.

Even fun events started to seem overwhelming to me. I had to accept that not all stress is caused by negative experiences. I was forced to reprioritize some of the more enjoyable aspects of my life too.

Cutting certain responsibilities and activities was easier for me after I was diagnosed. It was difficult for me to tell someone "no" before I was ill, but it was a lot easier afterward. This gave me the opportunity to focus on what was best for our family, which lowered my stress level. Since battling cancer quickly filled the time I had formerly devoted to other areas, I implemented the following coping techniques:

- *I Faced the Fire* by reading for understanding and to develop a battle plan. Cancer cells are no different from any other organism. *They have a strong desire to live*. But as I understood more about the disease and learned its weaknesses, the enemy became less intimidating. Knowledge was empowering and the possibility of overcoming the odds energized my spirit.
- *I Reframed the Problem*, which helped me think about cancer not as an all or nothing extreme, but as a different state of being. I made adjustments to my lifestyle, but did not go without anything I really wanted. I learned that cancer, which seemed like an ending, could be a positive event that came with many gifts if I thought of it that way. I had to change the way I adapted to my new life, and positive thinking cultivated a harvest of beautiful experiences.
- *I Implemented* what I learned, which lowered my stress level, and I felt better than I had in years. I hoped to eliminate cancer with every resource God gave me and fondly call the tools unveiled to me "My Daily Bread." It was as if He withheld the next piece of information until I was ready to receive it. Many of the changes I implemented made me feel better. And consequently, the stress subsided.
- *I Managed My Fears and Expressed Gratitude* by journaling and prayer. I belonged to support groups, and they were instrumental in helping me understand the technical aspects of the disease. But honestly, my main emotional support came from quiet times with God. And because of this, I am grateful for the personal relationship I have with Him.

Victim or Empowered, I Had a Choice

ME

Books on the subject of chronic illness, especially cancer and heart disease, suggest that most of these illnesses are "lifestyle diseases." The Standard American Diet tempts us every day by glamourizing convenience, taste, and price. Achievement and success, as defined by society, exhausts us, as our bodies try to neutralize the damage from unprecedented environmental factors. The result is that our immune systems have to work overtime to try to keep up. If they don't, we become vulnerable to a host of possible ailments.

If we are tempted to pursue the American dream and neglect our bodies and spirits, who says we do not have the power to reverse the cycle? We are perfectly made by God, and our bodies have the ability to repair themselves. Along with the advances in modern medicine, we can also support our immune systems with proper nutrition and a positive spirit. We should not simply wait and pray for God to heal us, but we can listen to what the universe is suggesting we do to achieve our goal of wellness. When I meet people who are hesitant to act, it reminds me of the story Moses told Joshua in the movie "The Ten Commandments":

There was a man whose house was threatened by a flood. When his neighbor left he said he should come with him. "No, he said, "I am waiting for God's help." The water kept rising. A man on a camel called to him, "Jump on," he said. "Save yourself!" "No, I'm waiting for God's help." The water rose to his roof. A man in a boat came by. He refused to get in it. "I'm waiting for God's help!"

He drowned. He was very angry when he came face to face with God. "Why didn't you save me!" he asked. God said, "I sent you the neighbor, I sent you the camel, and I sent you the boat. *What More Did You Want?"*

This story serves as a reminder that God doesn't physically or spiritually heal us by luck or accident. But rather He is a Father whose quiet voice guides His children to accept the help that the world has to offer. Cancer doesn't change that.

After watching this movie I realized I was waiting on the Lord, when in fact He was waiting on me! Once I acted on His guidance, the quality of my life became rich and beautiful again, especially when I recognized the greatest tool used by the enemy is discouragement. Because with this crippling emotion, he tried to suggest that my circumstances with cancer should become my god and the focus of my life. I am thankful for the day I grasped that discouragement got me nowhere; I had to act and trust in the Lord.

From "Why Me?" to "It's Not About Me!"

ME

I love this question! At first I asked the question expecting to learn what I had done to stress my immune system. But I decided to put a more positive twist on the question. Now, the "Why me?" answers are beautiful possibilities like:

- This is an opportunity to glorify God and be a testimony to His healing.
- My purpose is to teach others, through my words and actions, about the power of coping and adapting to a new lifestyle.
- Cancer is a reminder to reprioritize a hectic life; no one knows what tomorrow may bring.
- It's my chance to remind people: Today is beautiful! (When I had no hair and people knew I just received chemo, this was a fun phrase to use. Most looked at me with a puzzled facial expression.)
- Show others by example that it's possible to work and remain active through treatment.

Basically, I grew to accept that cancer was certainly not a matter of "Why me" nor was it even *about me*. The experience was more about how the effect of my actions rippled out and impacted the lives of others. It was Matthew 5:14-16, New International Version (NIV) that unveiled the truth:

You are the light of the world. A town built on a hill cannot be hidden. Neither do people light a lamp and put it under a bowl. Instead they put it on its stand, and it gives light to everyone in the house. In the same way, let your light shine before others, that they may see your good deeds and glorify your Father in heaven.

As a survivor of a chronic illness I recognize I have a slight advantage. When I allow my light to shine before others, it radiates brighter than it did in the past. Simply living each day with a positive attitude is a testimony to God's grace. I did not have to do anything extraordinary.

Once the shock from the initial diagnosis subsided, I realized my spirit was restless. I believe that God was stirring me up inside telling me there was something I was supposed to do. He wanted my light to shine. At first, I started a scrapbook to record my journey. I still felt restless. I wrote in a journal. I felt better but still restless. I decided to publish what I learned, and that turned out to be the answer. I finally found peace in purpose. I started dreaming of the possibility that I was saved to inspire others. Wow! But all this was easier as an aspiration than reality. To achieve my goal, I had to rise above the influence of my inner voices.

It was easy to become enslaved by negative thinking. Some of my thoughts attempted to trap and alienate me from the voice of God. Other thoughts, which I believed came from the devil, worked against God's voice and yearned to write a different ending to my story. I constantly battled thoughts like, "Why would you want to write a book, if you only have months to live?" "What makes you qualified to write a book?" "You are a numbers person, not a writer." "Your purpose is family and work." And by prayer, I persevered in spite of such thoughts.

Note: Some cancer survivors seem to work less or choose to not remain employed. If so, consider taking this time to impact the lives of others. It can be uplifting to your soul and as simple as taking an hour a week to volunteer.

The analogy of a rock being thrown into a body of water illustrates the impact of our actions. When we throw a little pebble into water, the ripple effect is not very noticeable. However, when we throw a larger rock into water the ripples are larger and extend out farther and farther from the source. I continually ask myself first, if I am satisfied with the size of the impact I am making, and second, if my actions have the potential to influence the lives of others with ripples that extend to people I may never meet. While constantly reminding myself, regardless of how much fuel is left in my lamp, it does not mean I have little or no light to shine. There is still a lot to offer!

At first I reluctantly accepted writing as my purpose, which originated at the point where my burden, passion and skills intersected. But in the end, I was grateful for the experience that was fueled by God's gift of perseverance.

The Word Was Peace

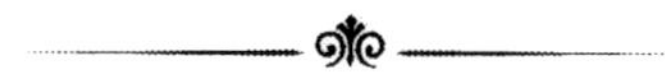

ME

I found peace, strength, and understanding in the Bible the day I purchased my first copy. I discovered the "Word" offered more than the "world" did. The devotional Bible proved to be an excellent choice for me, because it was already divided into 365 sections of daily reading. I loved the structure, and felt that the one-year goal of reading the entire Bible was attainable. And the daily devotions, short stories submitted by others, helped reinforce the passages I read each day. Since I was a spiritual rookie, the viewpoints expressed in these devotions provided a modern-day perspective that I could easily relate to. The Bible grounded my emotions and allowed me to realize my purpose in the midst of uncertainty.

There were many different Bibles at the Christian bookstore other than the daily devotional Bible. For those who appreciate order, there are chronologically written ones. There are also Bibles tailored for women, men, teenagers, or children. Although there are times when I prefer the New Living Translation version, I learned from the clerk that the New International Version is easier to read.

To my surprise, the Bible is not only a spiritual handbook, but also a guide for our physical body. Since I had never heard a sermon on how God intended for us to eat, I assumed the written word was only about right and wrong. Perhaps church could be a great place to start a grassroots effort to change the way Americans view nutrition. If Christians changed their eating habits to match God's intended plan and shared their testimonies, then others might follow.

Note: While I was on this crusade to find peace, all the paths originating from worldly answers seemed rather shallow and extremely cumbersome to me. But the Bible provided comfort, and I looked forward to reading the passage for the day. It was imperative that I find my own path, and the Bible was mine. Yours may be meditation, yoga, guided imagery, martial arts, or deep-breathing exercises. The possibilities are endless; make it your own. Our spiritual journey should bring comfort and contentment, not another daily task.

WAY It's important for people to find their own spiritual path, but there are a few moments of my own journey that I want to share. Just as meeting Chet (described in the introduction to Part II) gave me a blessed assurance, so did scripture at the times when I needed it most. Looking back in my journal, these events seem like part of a beautifully played masterpiece. I just didn't realize how it all fit together at the time.

My relationship with God encompasses a great deal of my life. But, for now, I'm going to describe two specific stories which demonstrate what my husband and I fondly called "coincidences." Two Bible passages reassured me that He is not just with me in good times. He is with me all the time. The day before my chemotherapy started, my devotional reading was Joshua 1:9 (NIV), "Do not be afraid; do not be discouraged, for the Lord your God will be with you wherever you go."

This reading definitely uplifted my spirits. My journal account of that day noted that "My blood pressure was 121/79, which is pretty good for receiving news about a Stage IV diagnosis." I recall receiving the news not with tears, but with optimism. This passage helped me relax and stay focused. I was ready to battle cancer and I did not feel alone, not even for one second.

In November of 2010, my first PET scan after five months of chemotherapy showed no evidence of disease. My reading for that day was from Isaiah 14:32 (NIV), "The Lord has established Zion and in her his afflicted people will find refuge." Coincidentally, the cancer facility where I received treatment is in Zion, Illinois.

The clean PET scan came the day before Thanksgiving. I could not have been more thankful for anything in my life. Even though I felt as though God had healed me before I even received the results, I was still anxious for the world to confirm the belief I already held in my heart.

While walking through the halls of the clinic hours before the results, an employee was singing "Give Thanks." I still see her frequently, but have not heard her sing in the hallways since. I often wondered if the song was meant for me to hear. The lyrics that warmed my heart that day are, "Give thanks with a grateful heart, Give thanks to the Holy One; Give thanks because He's given Jesus Christ, His Son (sung twice). And now let the weak say, 'I am strong,' let the poor say, 'I am rich,' Because of what the Lord has done for us (sung twice) Give Thanks!" Once I received the confirmation that God had taught me how to overcome insurmountable odds, I knew I had to share my story. That night I decided to write, not only to help others, but to also give thanks and glory to God.

The day I sat down to write the initial draft of this section, I attended a sermon that spoke of "mountaintop experiences." I realized in the past I had only allowed myself to feel God's grace in the good times. My mountaintop experiences were the times I stood in awe at places like the Grand Canyon, Zion National Park, Turkey Run State Park, Sebago Lake, and the Caribbean.

But then there were the times I dropped to my knees to face uncertainty or, in my case, my own mortality. God called me to follow at those times too, not just the good ones. It was easy for me to recognize and appreciate His splendor when I was viewing the sunset over the Grand Canyon with my sisters. However, I also had to learn how to cherish this relationship while I was sick from chemotherapy. How I followed Him determined the quality of my life. God was not just there in these mountaintop times, but He was there every time.

"People see God every day; they just don't recognize Him."
- Pearl Bailey

"She found her knees."
- My husband

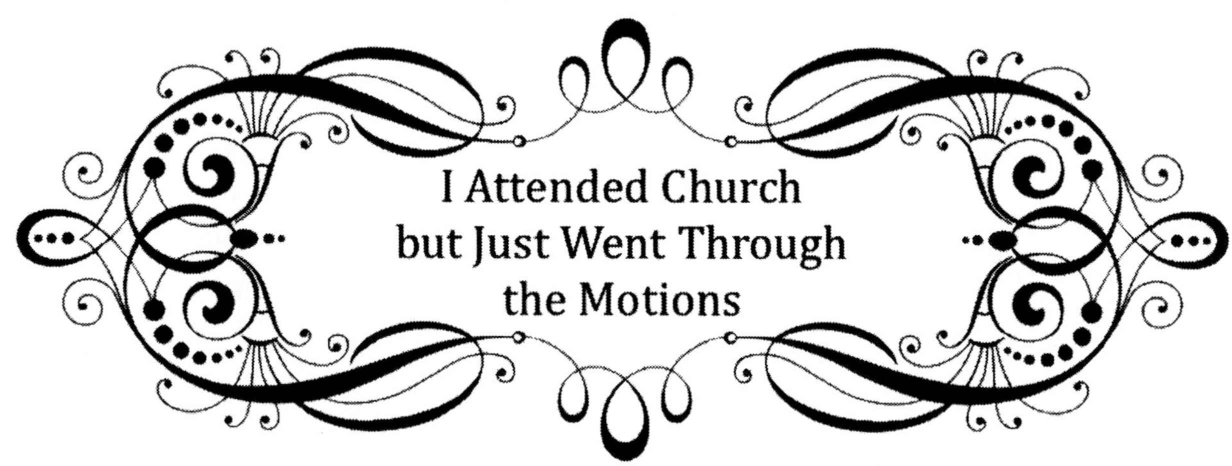

I Attended Church but Just Went Through the Motions

When I was first diagnosed, one of our credit union board members came to my office to visit. We shared our struggles and fears concerning our health. She left for about five minutes and walked back in my office. She said, “God told me to give this to you.” It was not just *any* Bible. It was *her* personal Bible. What a powerful gift. If she had just given me any Bible, I am not sure I would have been as receptive or taken the time to read it. But she gave me her own Bible, which inspired me to read and learn. She marked two passages that helped her through tough times. I waited to read it until I got home that afternoon eagerly anticipating the message. I crawled in bed to read the two passages. The first one, Isaiah 58:5-9, King James Version, read:

5. Is it such a fast that I have chosen? a day for a man to afflict his soul? is it to bow down his head as a bulrush, and to spread sackcloth and ashes under him? wilt thou call this a fast, and an acceptable day to the Lord?

6. Is not this the fast that I have chosen? to loose the bands of wickedness, to undo the heavy burdens, and to let the oppressed go free, and that ye break every yoke?

7. Is it not to deal thy bread to the hungry, and that thou bring the poor that are cast out to thy house? when thou seest the naked, that thou cover him; and that thou hide not thyself from thine own flesh?

8. Then shall thy light break forth as the morning, and thine health shall spring forth speedily: and thy righteousness shall go before thee; the glory of the Lord shall be thy rereward.

9. Then shalt thou call, and the Lord shall answer; thou shalt cry, and he shall say, Here I am. If thou take away from the midst of thee the yoke, the putting forth of the finger, and speaking vanity;

The passage speaks of the light breaking through like the morning. When I got to the end of the reading, the light coming into our bedroom was warm, pure, and glowing, like it was not of this world. Its temperature and beauty was perfection. And not only did the verses intrigue me, but the warmth of the light physically poured the message directly into my soul.

I got the chills, and I knew at that point my life was headed in a different direction. I simply needed to start walking in the course He set for me—and not the path of my choosing. I put it all in His hands and affirmed it out loud too. I cried tears of relief—like an enormous burden that was not mine to bear any longer was lifted from my shoulders.

Isaiah 53 was the other Bible passage marked by my friend, but it took me almost two years to fully appreciate the message. How beautiful are the gifts that we hold close to our heart? Then something happens to unleash them and they blossom with life months and months later. Days after she gave me her Bible, I wrote both passages on paper and taped them to the mirror that I use every day to get ready for work. I recited them out loud at quiet moments, but their full meaning remained unclear to me. As prayer is like a seed so was God's word. I was not ready to fully comprehend all that lay ahead of me, but I did have faith that someday I would truly understand.

That time came during the evening that I spoke the reading for the Good Friday church service. In five years I had read for our service twice. What are the odds the scripture would include the same passages given to me months before? Embedded in my reading for the night was Isaiah 53:4-5 (NIV):

Surely he took up our pain and bore our suffering, yet we considered him punished by God, stricken by him, and afflicted. But he was pierced for our transgressions, he was crushed for our iniquities; the punishment that brought us peace was on him, and by his wounds we are healed.

Over seven hundred days later I realize this passage was given to me so that I would finally understand that Jesus was brutally chastised for me! He died for me! He washed away all the daily sins I had committed against my body—my poor food choices, my stressful lifestyle, my poor attitude.

He took all that! And because I had faith I became strong and He gave me peace. He was whipped so I could be healed. God laid the weight of my sins on Jesus. And when I released and confessed them, I was free. Sweet, sweet freedom.

Solitude

ME

The voice of God was constantly speaking to me, and trying to get my attention. To hear the voice (some call it a gut feeling) I had to slow down, tune out the world, and just be with Him. Without distractions and realizing that God was rarely in the obvious, I was able to focus on His plan for me. I know He was with me all the time, but it was too easy to let life distract me from the relationship we both yearned for. Now that I decided to make it a priority, when I had a big decision to make, I received direction in silence. I accomplished this by finding a quiet place to pray or by walking in the country with my dog, because making a decision with the world buzzing around me was virtually impossible.

WAY There was one time in particular that I remember making a decision in solitude that ended up being a huge turning point in my treatment. It was at the beginning of the journey and I had not yet decided between the treatment options offered by the oncologist in my hometown. My spirit was restless. I needed time to ask God for guidance. So, I told my coworkers to expect me a few hours late. I went to the park and just sat there to think and listen. Something told me to call Cancer Treatment Centers of America.

Knowing that this cancer facility was a private organization made my mind race with the fear that, because of my health insurance plan, I may be told "No." A crippling, little word that had the potential to pack a punch loaded with even more disappointment and discouragement. How much more could I take? Even though my apprehension was stoked by evil inner voices, at the very least I needed to find out if this facility was a viable option.

I drummed up twenty seconds of courage to make the call, and I am glad I did. Within two hours I was their patient, my insurance was verified, our hotel reservations were made, and I had renewed hope. Peace showered over me after that day in the park. I had no doubt I was on the right path, but I am not sure I could have figured it out by rushing around with work and family. Sometimes I just have to stop, pray, and listen.

ME

I also found direction while I walked, got a massage, took a shower, or woke in the middle of the night; solitude was the common factor. These were the times that God provided guidance, because I was not distracted. In fact, the organization of this book actually came to me during a massage appointment. I was struggling with the decision to make the format seem more like a "how to" or like a "how would you?" I found the answer to that question in silence, and now Fight4u2 has the structure that matched its intended purpose.

When I prayed in the middle of the night for God's direction, He ministered to me in a special way. I gave my fears to God in the silence of the night and in return He gave me peace and understanding.

I have a sacred space in my bedroom for prayer that also represents the physical location for my time with God. It reminds me of my memories of when I was young and played tag. It is my spiritual home base, and it makes me feel safe and temporarily released from the weight of the world. When I was a child, all my tension released when I was able to make it to "home" before anyone tagged me. By making a place like that in our bedroom, I created a spiritual foundation. I use a piece of furniture that is a family heirloom. On the table, I put all the trinkets and pictures that bring me peace. This is where I kneel to pray at night in solitude.

Some clergy recommend finding a totally dark and quiet place completely free of distractions. Regardless of where you choose, keep in mind the times in the Bible when Jesus used solitude to prepare for trying times or to repair and recharge His soul afterward. For me, the passage that comes to mind is the chapter 14 of Matthew in which He feeds five thousand people with five loaves of bread and two fish. Part of verse 23 (NIV) reads, "After he had dismissed them he went up on a mountainside by himself to pray." Because Jesus existed in human flesh, He serves as the perfect role model and reminder of the importance of solitude and spending quality time with God.

Gratitude

ME

In the beginning, blending gratitude and cancer seemed as impossible as mixing oil and water. Although people who beat advanced-stage cancer and thrive oftentimes cultivate an attitude of gratitude, I was reluctant to believe that life was so delightful. In the midst of biopsies, surgical options, and scans, everything seemed less than wonderful, and I certainly did not feel up to appreciating it.

But if gratitude could help others conquer the beast called cancer, I had to try too. So, I started with small baby steps by noticing the little things. For me, it was sunsets and watching our crops break ground in the spring. I sat in awe of thousands of one-inch-high plants with the potential to mature to over ten feet tall. On one hand the corn was so little and vulnerable, but on the other hand it lined up in perfect little rows of promise. For the first time I truly admired the splendor of our farm, and the experience reminded me of the first time I fed my baby sister chocolate pudding. From the look on her face I could tell it was spectacular! By accident, I learned to be grateful by admiring the small stuff. And what I formerly took for granted became magnificent.

I developed a higher level of gratitude by writing in a journal. I was surprised to notice that very few of my entries were about the dark, deep emotions that I expected to pour out of me. More often I wrote about the parts of the day I wanted to recall later because I was thankful. So, I decided to take my "grateful mania" to new heights by ending every journal entry with at least three things that brought me pleasure. In the beginning most of the lists included something as simple as a great meal or a sunset, but at least I was recognizing something positive about my life.

As I look back, those initial entries were not deep or spiritual. Even with the first entry, dated June 6, 2010, about forty-five days from diagnosis, I could tell I was grasping to find something positive about the day. I was thankful for

- My husband and I setting up the radio under the kitchen cabinets,
- A great chicken and tomato dish,
- The sunset that showed up pink on dark clouds.

Frankly, I am rather embarrassed by my first attempts at expressing gratitude. But hopefully these raw, real-life examples can inspire others to express themselves even when times are tough. It was an emotion that I had to relearn. Don't be surprised if it takes practice.

It was apparent I was becoming more open to the therapeutic benefits of recording gratefulness. Within two weeks of that first entry, I was recognizing the beauty in life again. Even though I was enduring the stress of multiple scans, on June 18, 2010, I was thankful for

- The picture of Lake Sebago (the location of my childhood memories) that popped up on my husband's phone before the scan,
- Scan technician's name was the same as my dad's,
- Quiong instructor's last name was the same as my sisters (Quiong is an exercise and healing technique developed in China),
- The blueberries I ate for breakfast were so good, and they reminded me of Maine,
- My mind/body therapist reminded me of a close friend.

The entries revealed a glimmer of gratitude, and I seemed open to the possibility that life was still pleasant and comforting.

Then, one month after that entry, my journal shows that I was definitely getting back on track. From my first entry, which seemed like it was written by a child, to this last one, it was apparent that I knew where I needed to start giving thanks and praise. On July 14, I was grateful for

- News of the decline of my tumor markers, the indicators in my blood work that detected the extent of my disease,
- My first prayer from the heart. It was from me, not recited from a book, and as a result, I physically felt His love pour over me.

TRI The power of gratitude eventually shifted over to our family life too. A year later after a trip to Florida we held hands in a circle and each person shared something about our experience that they enjoyed. We called it COG "circle of gratitude" time. Some of the responses were humorous. But it was also rewarding to see our children recall experiences that most would categorize as trivial, and it helped us understand what constituted memorable events for our family.

In that same year, which was 2011, was the first holiday we had our Grateful Christmas Tree. There were no traditional lights, balls, tinsel, garland or ornaments. Instead our family gathered items that represented events over the year we were thankful for. We hung pictures of family trips, my scan results, medals, certificates, awards and ticket stubs. On the top, as our star, was a homemade cross with Jesus written down the center. The tree was not a chore. There was no digging stuff out of storage, and it took about 15 minutes. The kids said over and over again this was their favorite tree ever. It was so rewarding to see the pride they had in our one-of-a-kind creation when visitors came over.

After we took our keepsakes off the tree I laid them out together and took a picture of all the items. Since then our family tradition has been to have a Grateful Tree for Christmas, and the picture collage is a great way to look back and remember the gifts our family received from year to year.

Destiny Was Between God and Me

ME

No one ever gave me a timeline. I did not ask, nor did it come up in conversation. I never got on the internet looking for it. I knew my mother turned to the web for the answers about my prognosis. And I could tell by her spirit, that I did not want to do the same. I believed no one on this earth had the authority to tell me how long I had to live, and that my will was stronger than anyone's educated guess. There were no material facts to substantiate the exact path of my prognosis, and I certainly did not want to plan my future based on the world's expectations.

My optimism did not stop at disregarding a statistical timeline. For some reason people with Stage IV cancer are not expected to work. When I called about my disability insurance for the surgery, my representative asked how many weeks I expected to be off for chemotherapy. I was shocked she asked. And she was equally surprised by my response that I intended to keep working. She told me that she worked claims for many people across the nation, and I was only the second advanced-stage cancer patient she knew who kept working.

My husband also supported my efforts to fulfill my own expectations. He has a family member who worked in healthcare, and she wanted to warn me ahead of time of all the side effects that I might experience from the chemotherapy. Her intentions were good and intended with a loving spirit. And like a good girl scout, she felt I needed to be equipped to handle all the possibilities. My husband sternly said, "No, she will figure it out on her own." He knew I had done a lot of preparation and was set on a path of positive expectations. I expected to continue to work. I expected to eat a healthy diet. I expected to walk with my dog and play volleyball with my friends. I expected to be a part of our children's activities. I expected to keep my life as normal as possible.

My husband knew I had planted this seed of optimism, and he protected me from succumbing to the cancer patient stereotype. He knew if my beliefs were misguided and unrealistic, we could adapt as needed. We approached this with the attitude that it was more beneficial for me to have high expectations and make adjustments, than to miss out on living the life I still longed for. I'd rather fall seven times and get up eight, than not take a step.

Worry Was Like a Rocking Chair. It Kept Me Busy but Got Me Nowhere.

ME

What an awesome gift I received the day I listened to a sermon that reminded me that almost 90 percent of what we waste time worrying about one, will never happen, two, has already happened and cannot be changed, or three, are situations beyond our control.

That leaves less than 10 percent for us to worry about that we could have influence over.

Soon after I was diagnosed I'm sure I was concentrating on the 90 percent and not focusing on how to properly manage the 10 percent I had some control over. My life's decisions were tainted with worry and sorrow, and these emotions that looped in my head, like a dog chasing its own tail, provided no answers and drained energy from the day. I had to learn to look at things differently and remember that even though I wasn't guaranteed tomorrow, I still felt great today!

I was so thankful that I stumbled across this insight and reevaluated how I was spending my time emotionally. If I had spent precious moments worrying about dying, I would have missed out on trips to Arizona, Florida, Texas, and Las Vegas. I was going through treatment every three weeks, but it proved to be one of the most memorable years of my life.

When my mind started wandering, usually in the middle of the night, I either prayed for God to take the worry from me, or I said the following phrase, written by author Greg Anderson, over and over until the negative thoughts subsided: "I am cancer-free, a picture of health, thank you God." In his book, *Cancer: 50 Essential Things to Do,* he claimed this affirmation helped save his life. Greg says, "I changed my health with one very powerful affirmation. Right in the middle of the cancer battle, starting at the point where I was down to 112 pounds, confined to bed, and on morphine to control the pain, I began to affirm: 'I am cancer-free, a picture of health. Thank you God.'" He said this up to 500 times per day, and his health miraculously improved.

TRI

<u>Other suggestions for affirmations that may work well are:</u>

- Thank you, God, for giving me a long and fulfilling life.
- Every day I am getting stronger and healthier.
- I am a child of God, worthy of His best.
- The Lord is My Shepherd.

Note: I found it helpful to take pictures of written affirmations and scripture by adding them to the lock screen on my smart phone, because it reminded me to recite them multiple times throughout the day. My personal favorite was Jeremiah 29:11 (NIV) "'For I know the plans I have for you,' declares the Lord, 'plans to prosper you and not to harm you, plans to give you hope and a future.'"

ME

I started my mornings with a positive statement. For months, when I woke up, the absolute first thing that popped in my head was "I have cancer." For the most part, after I had decided to be more positive, this was still the first thought that I thought each morning, but I quickly followed it up with Psalm 118:24 (NLT), "This is the day the Lord has made, we will rejoice and be glad in it."

The Bible teaches us in Matthew 6:34 (NIV), "Therefore do not worry about tomorrow, for tomorrow will worry about itself. Each day has enough trouble of its own." When I got wrapped up in my "what if" feelings, I missed out on the present. I discovered that trying to figure out tomorrow did me absolutely no good, and it slowed me down. Worry allowed a satanic, crippling factor into my life, but I found that the word of God strengthened me.

I was comforted when the pastor said, "May the Lord bless you and keep you and give you peace that surpasses all understanding." At first I only found comfort, but now I also understand it. The Bible teaches us in Philippians 4:6 (NIV), "Do not be anxious about anything, but in every situation, by prayer and petition, with thanksgiving, present your requests to God." When I sincerely acknowledged my anxiety and came before God in the right spirit of thankfulness and asked Him to lift it from my heart, the result was peace. I had the blessings of peace that surpassed all understanding. The feeling was indescribable. It came from faith, not from trying to figure it out.

Released the Past

ME

I, like most cancer patients, could look back on my life prior to diagnosis and identify a major stressor in my life. For me it was a stressful career and placing other people's needs before my own. I also had unresolved issues from my past. There were decisions I felt guilty about, and I asked God for forgiveness, not only for myself but others. There was nothing I could do about the past. So, I had to learn how to trade in my fierce judgment of myself and others for feelings of compassion.

When my past was holding me back from believing I deserved a future, I turned to Isaiah 1:18 (NLT): "'Come now, let's settle this,' says the Lord. 'Though your sins are like scarlet, I will make them as white as snow. Though they are red like crimson, I will make them as white as wool.'"

Harboring resentment toward others was also crippling my spirit. Greg Anderson's book *Cancer: 50 Essential Things to Do* offered a simple phrase for forgiveness. "(Name), I totally and completely forgive you. I release you to the care of God. I affirm your highest good."

I realized that by holding grudges against those who had wronged me, my spirit was damaged, but it was not beyond repair. I simply had to turn those bad feelings over to God and know that He had the power to handle them. When I was living in despair from others' actions, I may have well been poisoning myself. Dwelling on those past circumstances did nothing to enhance my today. Furthermore, the wrongdoers were off living the life of their dreams or better yet may have not even realized the extent of my pain. And I am pretty sure they were not losing any sleep over any of it, even though I was.

If I found myself thinking about something that made me fearful or angry, it was helpful to write these thoughts on paper and then physically destroy them by burning or shredding the paper, thereby declaring that these thoughts no longer served me. I am not sure if it was the act of physically writing it down (not on a computer but with pencil and paper), or if it was the destruction of what I wrote, but healing came as a result. And I was finally able to forgive.

Chapter Four
A Light That Breaks Forth Like the Dawn

I Admired the Donut, Not the Hole

ME

It took me a while, but I transitioned toward living a more fulfilling life by continually setting positive and attainable goals for myself—goals like walking a certain amount of miles per week or looking forward to going away on trips—while striving to trust in God's will instead of wasting time worrying. Because when I allowed worry to cripple my life experiences, I realized I was focusing on the hole (cancer) and not admiring the donut (life).

I found I wanted to travel more, so that my busy, task-oriented life could not consume all my days. After each trip I usually made plans for the next excursion. It could be something as simple as scheduling a weekend with friends. The point was that I had something to look forward to. In 2011, I traveled to four other states. More than likely, I would not have set aside the time to go on these trips if I had not been diagnosed with cancer. The diagnosis forced me to reevaluate how I spent my time.

Almost one year to the day after my grim prognosis, which at the time made it seem strange to look to the future, I recorded five goals in my journal. I wondered if my purpose was migrating away from managing the credit union to helping fellow survivors discover ways to enhance their life. It is the only time I have actually written down my goals. I am extremely task oriented, but I had not written down ambitions on a piece of paper before. I guess time will tell if they come true. Although as I wrote them I felt, "This is crazy, but what if? What if these goals all became reality? How fulfilling my life could be!"

My Journal Entry 4-13-11

"This is the Day" [a song by the group The The] your life will surely change. All the signs are pointing to that. At the [Illinois Credit Union] annual convention the keynote speaker said to write down your goals, commit to them, and take action. Then the powers of the universe take you in that same direction. I feel it. Last night, that song [by The The] was on when I saw a shooting star in the sky. Thank you, Lord. This morning the tag of my coffee said, "Grace brings contentment." Thank you, Lord. So, what if? What if I write a book on my journey and help others like me? And the credit union is not my path but helping survivors is? I want people to discover that cancer can be beautiful, rewarding, and actually an act of love from God—an act that gets you on track—a track of passion and purpose.

<u>My Goals: (from the same journal entry dated 4-13-11)</u>

1. Write the book to help others pick and choose what strengthens them
2. Publish it – donate half to holistic research for cancer
3. Present at speaking engagements
4. Quit the credit union (I am thinking really big here)
5. Tell the world about my testimony sitting with Matt Lauer [host of the Today Show on NBC]

So, I wrote down my goals and trusted in God's plan for me—the plan He had weighed on my heart.

My fondest memory for remembering how awesome the donut is and not focusing on the hole was an occasion I shared with my husband. It was Halloween of 2010. And we had just celebrated our one-year wedding anniversary, when we had the opportunity to dress up for a costume party. Since my husband is mostly bald and so was I, we decided to switch places in celebration of our anniversary. He wore my wedding dress, wig, and veil. I wore a suit, tie, and no wig.

I had a little bit of hair left on my head. So, to prepare for the evening, we cut the top totally bald and left the sides longer to mimic my husband's. While we were in the shower with the trimmers, we laughed so hard that we cried. He kept saying, "I can't look at you!" That night I snickered to myself before I fell asleep. I figured I was the only girl in the world that intentionally cut her hair bald on top and left it longer around the sides. We sent pictures to close family and friends. They thought we photo-shopped the picture, and we had to assure them it was real.

In Giving, I Received

ME

Love is not a noun but a verb. I have been called a generous, thoughtful person for the most part. But when I was diagnosed, I reevaluated how much I considered others' needs. Perhaps it was the fear of facing my Maker and not being sure I led the best life that I could have? Nevertheless, I knew I could not take my money with me. Granted I could have left a larger nest egg for my family, but I decided I would rather experience firsthand how my gifts from God could impact other people's lives. So, I stepped up my giving to 10 percent of my income.

The first thing I noticed, to my surprise, is that, for the first time in my life, I didn't worry about money. I didn't toil over if a donation was too little or too much. The weirdest coincidence was that when I gave, oftentimes I received a check in the mail the same day. I felt as though I had more money than ever before. Best of all, money was not the driving force of my decisions anymore. What a gift—to be released from the bondage of the almighty dollar.

I also stepped up my volunteering for local and global efforts. Cancer afforded me the opportunity to reprioritize my time, and I chose to ground myself with service. Soon after diagnosis, I was asked to serve on our Stewardship Committee at church. As a congregation we assembled school kits, healthcare kits, and meals for people overseas—which were all very rewarding projects. But I share a journal entry to show that sometimes giving was not always planned out ahead of time. I also became more open to spontaneous opportunities as well.

<u>My Journal Entry Dated, 12-8-11</u>

Come near to God and he will come near to you. James 4:8a (NIV)

As Christmas approaches I start scouring the stores for deals. It helps that I walk the malls for exercise, but nonetheless it is still difficult to find bargains weeks before the holiday season. I had gone to a national chain that carries children's clothes and found items for $1.97 plus 35 percent off. I was pretty proud of the four oversized shopping bags of items for under $100 that I was able to donate to a local organization.

I walked back in the same store two days later to find a picked-over rack of items under two dollars. I left the store, continued walking and a thought popped in my head. What if they sold me everything that was left for an additional discount? I hesitated at the store entrance for a moment and then noticed two ladies working together at the front of the store. I thought to myself, this is my chance. I am going in!

I shared my offer with them to take the remaining items for a donation. Without hesitation they simply responded, "Give us 15-20 minutes, and we will pull items from the entire store."

Of course, at that point my charge card started to quiver. So, I asked, "How much for the items?" They responded once again without hesitation, "Forty seven cents per item." I wanted to drop to my knees at that moment and thank God for moving me to simply ask. It ended up being less than two hundred dollars for about five hundred items. I forgot to mention that I asked about an additional 10 percent for using my store credit card, which they also agreed to without hesitation. I figured I was on a roll. So I might as well ask.

But the story does not end there, I was thinking to myself, while they were ringing each item individually because they needed to be price adjusted. Why was this so easy? God gave me the answer.

In conversation while paying for the items the store manager asked me again, "What is this organization?" I went into a little more detail than in the previous conversation when I made my plea for support. I explained that this not-for-profit organization gets Christmas gifts to the needy families who miss out on receiving other assistance during the holidays.

She shared her story about how, one year, her dad was in a serious car accident and could not buy Christmas presents for them. She said some of his coworkers stepped up and bought each child a couple gifts. She said, "I will never forget that." There was my answer! God gave her a chance to experience what her father's coworkers did for her years earlier. That is why this was so easy. It was not my savvy shopping or persuasive request. It was God working through both of us to show us the beauty of giving.

Because of experiences like this, I learned the more I lovingly gave, the more my heart filled with joy. Sometimes thinking of others did not involve a lot of time, something as simple as gifts for my healthcare providers was uplifting. But during these times I had to resist the urge to say to the Lord, "Look what I did for you!" And remember that I was blessed with the experience, because of Him.

"Greatness is not found in possessions, power, position, or prestige. It is discovered in goodness, humility, service, and character."

- Unknown

Simplify

ME

In my original manuscript an entire chapter with multiple sections was devoted to simplicity. But during the rewrite I felt it was more appropriate to "simplify" it to a couple pages instead. So, with that in mind, here are some tips that made coping with cancer more manageable.

Care page. One of the best things I did for myself, friends, and loved ones, was to create a website that updated others on my progress. When I was first diagnosed, I found myself on the phone constantly. It took time to explain something that was so foreign to me. Plus, I had to determine how up-to-date each person was at the beginning of the conversation. Everything changed and progressed so quickly, I couldn't remember. Once I started the website, I updated it when I had time. In the beginning it was almost daily, and then it became a couple times a week. Now it's updated occasionally, but almost always after a doctor visit. It allows me to share information when I have the time, and likewise, my family and friends catch up when they have a free moment.

My employer developed my care page for me. But there are websites, such as www.mylifeline.org and www.carepages.com that provide the same kind of assistance. For people who are not technically savvy, a friend or relative can set this up. I knew patients who didn't even write their own posts. A family member did it for them. For me, this was about balancing what was best for me but still remembering that people cared. Leaving them in the dark was not a viable option and talking on the phone left me with hardly any free time. The webpage was truly a blessing for everyone.

The best benefit of the care page was that I could live a normal life while I was with my friends. I did not have to spend the first fifteen minutes of our visit talking about cancer, because they already knew what was happening.

Support Groups. I found support groups were helpful for gathering information, but not necessarily for uplifting my spirit. That is the reality of this disease, when we mourn together for our friends. Gathering with fellow patients is not for everyone, but I found it informative to learn from others like me. They helped me sort out the pros and cons of different surgical options and suggested organizations that offered support to me and my family. (A list of some of these organizations is recorded in the appendix.)

I am glad I gave it a chance. I learned by listening to others rather than by reading. I do believe we truly need each other to survive and thrive.

Setting Priorities. "When you say 'yes' to that which matters least, you are saying 'no' to what matters most."This quote by Rochelle Melander, author of *Write-A-Thon* helped me adjust my priorities. I was glad to use the cancer as an excuse to avoid responsibilities that I was not that crazy about. I especially loved that no one questioned me when I said, "I can't do this right now."

There were days when I left work a little early to take some time for myself without my conscience telling me otherwise. Cancer treatment provided the gift of "me-time" with less guilt. I grew to appreciate that an unplanned, unstructured afternoon was fun, and not every moment had to revolve around accomplishing a task.

As a family we started respecting the Sabbath Day more than we had in the past. Our family used to go, go, go constantly. Now, we have reserved this time for rest, hobbies and fellowship.

Lists, Lists and More Lists. I had pads of paper everywhere. My memory was extremely challenged during chemotherapy, which has been somewhat restored over time, but the process was slow. It was stressful for me to forget tasks that I might have to backtrack and do later. So, I made lists to help manage my day.

I knew even the lists were getting cumbersome when I looked at my reminders and the first item said, "see other list." But then I got a smart phone and downloaded a free app that electronically managed my different tasks. This technology was a time saver. I maintained lists for the day, remembered information for the book, saved questions for the doctor, and kept track of ideas for a church committee I served on.

The notes for the doctor were so helpful. I made the most of my appointments by having questions literally at my fingertips. I often started my list for my next appointment as soon as I left the last one. Between appointments, I documented any changes, symptoms, and worries I noticed. Monitoring pain, numbness, digestion, sores, appetite, and energy helped my team of experts evaluate my treatment plan. Basically, I kept a journal about my body and highlighted its strengths and weaknesses for them. I didn't edit anything. I let my doctor decide what was important and what wasn't. Because I didn't want to hear the words, "I wish we had known that sooner."

Not only were the lists helpful during my doctor visits, but there were routine errands I had to accomplish at the hospital. I just checked items off my electronic list when they were completed and unchecked them in preparation for the next visit. The simple tasks of my life were organized in one spot. What a lifesaver. Before, I had felt like the kid with the grocery list from my mom, repeating "bread, milk, and sugar...bread, milk, and sugar..." until I arrived at the store. Now I just enter all the items on my phone and watch the beautiful sunset or sleep peacefully instead of worrying about being forgetful.

A Wingman to Doctor Appointments. I took family and friends, and once I even took a tape recorder. I needed someone or something listening other than me. Because of my preoccupied thoughts, my caregivers heard things that I did not recall. I was reluctant to take a recorder, but I wish I had done it more often. My sisters wanted to hear exactly what the doctor had to say when they could not be there.

A Binder, Hole Punch, and Dividers. I stored all my paperwork in one binder. I accumulated a lot of paperwork. And believe me, it got heavy! So, I recommend one with a built-in shoulder strap. I had sections separated with dividers for bills, test results, pathology reports, blood work, supplement lists, etc. This information was at my fingertips when needed, and it was easily transported.

I also keep blood work in chronological order on a spreadsheet. It was helpful to monitor trends. The binder made it easier to remain proactive by staying organized with information that was easily accessible.

It would have been a treat for me, if I had thought of organizing a cancer experience binder sooner. I could have compiled sections on cancer research, contacts, Bible verses, exercise, recipes, nutrition, supplements, etc. When I came across something interesting, I could have made a copy and kept it in my binder without having to search for it later. Sometimes I came across information that was interesting, but I was not ready to process it or take the time to read the entire article.

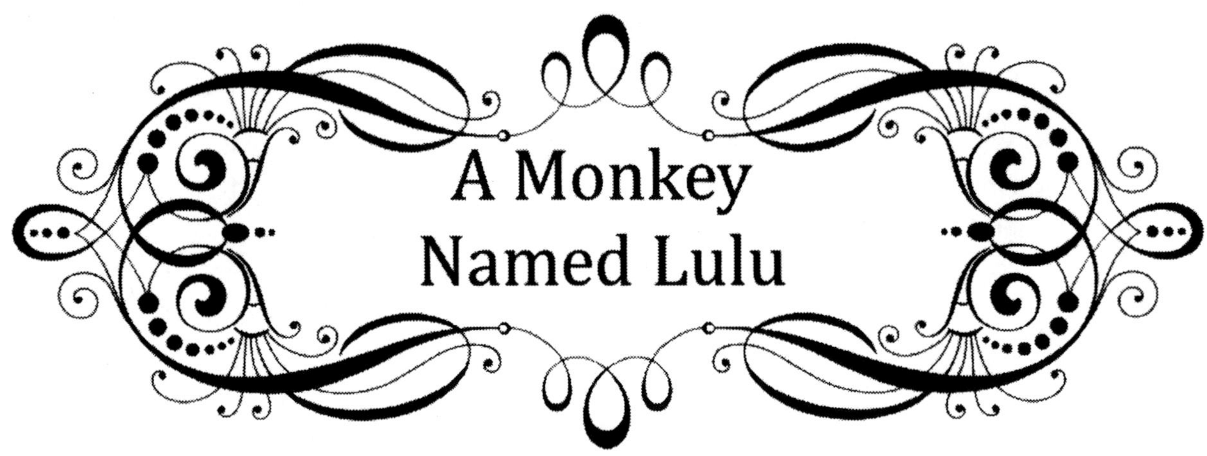

A Monkey Named Lulu

When the rough draft of this book was done, I started inquiring about publishing. For the most part, the people I asked indicated that it was difficult and expensive to get this accomplished. Feeling overwhelmed, I took a break from writing.

During this time my husband and I did some vacationing. On one trip, while waiting at the airport, I had the urge to stroll through the terminal. Since I was continually looking for new material to help facilitate the fight, I passed the time at the bookstore. I purchased a paperback called *The Happiness Project* by Gretchen Rubin. For some reason it took me a while to finish, but now I realize why. Much later, when I decided to continue reading it again, there were a series of events that beautifully unfolded as soon as the time was right.

At the beginning of that week I opened a fortune cookie that prepared me for what lay ahead. The message inside read "you will receive an unusual gift."

A couple days later I woke up in the middle of the night to read, which rarely happened anymore, because I usually slept well through the night. At three in the morning I decided to pick up Gretchen's book again and continue on. She told of a website, www.lulu.com, for self-publishing some of her memoirs, which rekindled my interest in getting this information compiled. I figured if there was a possibility that no one else would help me, I'd just publish the material myself.

That evening at Vacation Bible School clearly reaffirmed the intention of the gift I received the night before. Throughout the week the kids were introduced to different characters. These animals, called Bible Buddies, served as physical reminders of their message for the session that night. On that particular day the children were introduced to a monkey named Lulu, which happened to be spelled exactly the same as the website in the book I had read the night before. The caption under Lulu's picture read "God gives great gifts."

People Flooded Me with Ideas for Fighting Cancer

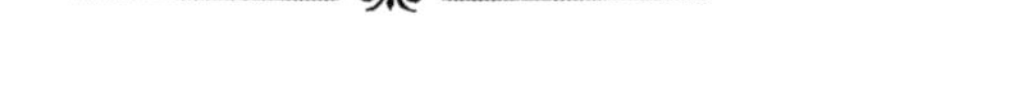

ME

A sermon I attended stated that we process approximately seven hundred thousand words a week! That is a lot to sort out. As a cancer patient, I can't help but wonder if I filtered out even more than that.

I received phone calls and visits from others about this or that miracle cure. Their intentions were good, BUT – yes, this is a big but – I still had to truly believe it benefitted me. After a while I realized that sometimes God worked through others to help me. But which information was guidance sent from above and delivered by a worldly messenger? The way I tried to filter the recommendations from others was to go with my "gut." There were some suggestions I was simply not comfortable with; they did not sit well with me. So, I'd tuck them away in my memory only to hear them resurface later in conversation with a different group of people. At that point I used the second-time rule. If I heard the same information more than once, then I would do further research.

One type of information I could not afford to filter out from the very beginning, was general breast cancer information. After my biopsy, I read a paperback book in my "breast cancer welcome packet" from our local clinic. It taught me the lingo of the disease. I valued this education, because it was imperative to learn the jargon in order to understand the doctors and my treatment options.

Even one year after diagnosis I was still caught off guard by this new language I was learning. I had just received the news that my scans were clear and posted the results on my blog. A friend of mine replied that they were so excited and could not believe I was NED. I snickered to myself and thought, "Who the heck is NED, and what has he done to me?" Turns out NED in the cancer world means "no evidence of disease." So, trust me I learned new lingo all the time. But especially in the beginning, I had to think of cancer fighting as a new career; there was a lot to learn in a short period of time. It was imperative that I speak the language.

Friendships

ME

This experience heightened my awareness that I had friends for a reason, a season, and a lifetime. As my life with cancer changed so did the people in each of these categories.

I had to ask myself whether my friends bring out my strengths or my weaknesses. Do they help me toward my goal of wellness or make it more challenging? I felt it was necessary to spend more of my free time with people who supported my lifestyle. I got involved with Bible study groups instead of going out to dinner and having drinks with friends. As much as it hurt, I had to stand among others who complemented my efforts and did not make them more challenging.

I learned that I needed to focus on who was there for me and not dwell on the ones that were not. I gratefully embraced the friendships I gained because of this experience. And I was amazed by the support I received from people I did not really know that well. The whole dynamic changed, which I welcomed, rather than fought by holding unrealistic expectations.

RE

Many acknowledge that friendships change after diagnosis. I think part of the reason is that our friends do not know what to say and may think that we need our privacy, but in actuality that is when we need them the most. Or our friends may try to protect us from activities they assume we would not engage in, rather than letting us exclude ourselves.

An article written by Laurie Wertich in the Cancer Fighters Thrive magazine (Spring, 2012) listed some communication guidelines to avoid with cancer patients. One might assume that this list is mostly for those who are caregivers, but strangely enough, I realized that even I have done a lot of these conversation no-no's.

- Don't use well-meaning but trite phrases such as, "Everything will work out" and "God has a plan."
- Don't say, "I know just how you feel" or "I understand." Unless you have endured the exact same thing, you really don't know how the person feels.
- Don't make comparisons such as "My Aunt Sally had cancer, and she had treatment X." Cancer comes in many varieties, and different people need different treatments. Let the doctors do the doctoring and instead focus on being a friend. (I cannot tell you how many times this happened to me, while I constantly reminded myself that every treatment and how each person handles it varied.)

- Don't trivialize the pain with such phrases as "It's just hair; it will grow back."
- Don't pity the patient.

So how do we shift to a more supportive conversation? The same article listed the following suggestions.

- Listen. Just simply listen with an open heart. Maintain eye contact and be present for your friend.
- Say, "I'm sorry you're going through this. I am here for you." And be there.
- Be natural. Treat your friend in the same way you always have.
- Maintain regular contact. Your friend may feel too tired or ill to socialize, but continue to check in and let him or her know you are there.
- Extend invitations to social events and let him or her say yes or no as appropriate. Social outings provide an opportunity to take a break from focusing on cancer. Your friend will appreciate the invitation even if he or she cannot attend. Don't exclude your friend.
- Incorporate humor when possible. Laughter can be very uplifting.
- Be specific. Rather than saying, "Let me know if there is anything I can do," say, "I have free time on Monday mornings; can I mow your lawn and pick up your groceries?"
- Make plans for the future. This gives your friend something to look forward to and also indicates that you plan on sticking around for the duration.
- Be positive and encouraging.

ME

There were many, but the most memorable moment of friendship was when one of my best friends drove four hours to sit with me during treatment. Of course, we made it an excursion with shopping and restaurant stops along the way, but I will never forget how her compassionate act will remain etched into my soul.

I was receiving a new type of infusion and experienced mild allergic reactions to the treatment, which included itchy skin and a prickly feeling in my upper lip. While they were giving me a dose of anti-allergy drugs, she leaned over and gently rested her hand on my forearm. She did not say anything; she was simply there for me.

Nothing Was Sacred

ME

Not only were my husband and I very open, but we also encouraged our children to share the news with their own friends. (At the time of diagnosis they were fourteen, eleven, and nine.) They were showered with support within hours. Their classmates and teammates signed cards to give me. The kids in Vacation Bible School organized a car wash to raise money for breast cancer. My daughter's softball team wore pink bracelets for their last game. Our youngest daughter attended a Pink Gymnastics Meet at The University of Illinois. As a guest coach for the event, she was on the floor with the squad for the entire meet.

Being free about our struggles with cancer opened the door for love from our community to flow into our lives. It was probably the best decision we made for our family. Everyone was incredibly supportive. Candidness brought compassion, not pity. It was uplifting to see our children's spirits raised by the love of others, as I witnessed the uncertainty in their eyes become trumped with benevolence.

I observed each of our children coping in different ways. Our oldest child came home and told us how her friends asked how we were doing. I could tell it meant a lot to her that they were interested. Our middle child was more attentive and helped me cook. And the youngest expressed her emotions with art, by incorporating little pink ribbons into pictures.

We used the word breast and cancer and did not try to call it something other than what it was. This may have been easier since our children were older, but nothing was taboo or sacred. We kept them informed of what to expect, and forewarned them of sickness, pain and hair loss.

The purpose of our open-door policy was initially about doing what we felt was best for our children, but I soon realized that it was also uplifting for me as well. I was blessed with cards, books, flowers, and sentimental gifts with Bible verses. I received gifts from members of the community that I had only met on occasion. Their thoughtfulness was unparalleled and helped fuel my expectations of the future.

Looking Good Was Not My Problem

ME

Probably one of the most frequent statements I hear is, "You look great!" Inside I snicker to myself, "Looking good has never been my problem." Even with no hair and side effects from chemotherapy treatments, I have made an extra effort to remain fashionable. The changes have even been noticeable to my friends. They could tell I had "stepped it up."

Since my diet had drastically changed, my body also changed, and I needed to adjust my wardrobe accordingly. And I enjoyed it! I strived to project strength in all facets of my life, which carried over in my style. I did not want to appear sick by sluffing around in yoga pants and sweatshirts, but rather seem as normal as possible. I guess, like my diet, my appearance was one more aspect of my life that I felt I had control over.

As my body changed I adapted and had fun with it, but what woman does not enjoy shopping? I had a blast "coping" with my new look. Here are some suggestions that helped me accomplish the task on a small budget:

Big Wardrobe for Small Change. We were blessed with the resources to go on shopping sprees every two months, but I chose to spend our money on family trips instead. So, I used unconventional means to achieve the same result. I found designer clothes at garage sales, thrift stores, and consignment shops. It took more time, but I enjoyed the challenge.

After migrating from a processed foods diet to a whole foods diet I lost weight pretty rapidly. Each time I changed sizes, I took my old clothes to a consignment shop, and I used the money I earned to purchase smaller ones. Living in the Midwest, I found garage sales to be a great option in the summer months. I often found brand name clothing for literally pennies on the dollar with the store tags still attached. Coincidentally, the weekend I wrote this section, I found a pair of tall-sized designer pants that had a forty-six dollar tag for a quarter.

After our garage sale season ended, I frequented thrift shops. Still using the money I made from the consignment shop, I found new treasures. Ironically, I received the most compliments on the clothing I purchased out of someone's yard or a thrift store. Not only were their responses funny when I confessed that my clothing came from a garage sale, but I also enjoyed the hunt and challenge of making a sharp looking outfit from these venues. Another bonus was feeling like I had my own little side business, because I was making money on my clothes by purchasing them for change, wearing them for a while, then selling them for dollars.

I Wondered How I Looked with Short Hair. I assumed I'd discover what I looked like with short hair when I reached my golden years. I never dreamed that the occasion would arise as a result of chemotherapy at forty years old. Nonetheless, I was still curious. So before my hair fell out, I went to the hairdresser for a short haircut. It was enjoyable to see the results with no regrets. Plus, when my hair fell out a week later, I had much shorter strands of hair to deal with all over the house. Once my hair was more than half gone, my husband clipped the rest off for me. Again I felt in control by cutting my own hair rather than allowing the cancer to take it from me. I took it in my own time.

I also tried on wigs before my hair fell out. I assumed it would be easier to fit me with a wig if the professional knew what I looked like before chemotherapy. My mom and sisters came and offered their opinion, and the stylist trimmed the wig to shape my face. After my hair fell out, I learned about the option of going to the American Cancer Society for assistance with a wig.

Oddly enough my favorite wig was from a local business that catered to African American women. Most of the selections were very reasonable, under $50.00. As soon as I walked in the store the clerk saw the look on my face as I gazed across a sea of black haired wigs. She assured me that certain selections came in blonde. The one I chose was $26.95.

Since I was open about my walk with cancer, it allowed me to wear several fun and different wigs. I ended up choosing ones that were black, red and blonde. I figured if everyone knew anyway, why limit myself to one look? I told my husband it was like he was married to all of Charlie's Angels.

As my hair grew back in I spiked it up with gel and sported the boy cut. I still wear it that way. Many people tell me they like it better than long hair, but I also appreciate the convenience. The part I love the most is that I have been able to give up hair care products, especially hair spray. All I use now is a dab of natural hair gel, and I am out the door. I think I spend less time on my hair now than I did with my wig, and I certainly spend less time than I did before cancer. It leaves more time for me, instead of for my vanity.

When my hair started growing back, strangers came up to me and complimented my hair style. I responded with a proud smile and replied, "Thanks, it is my one million dollar haircut." After a couple confused faces, I decided I should simply say thank you.

Note: I was surprised to find the synthetic wigs looked better than the ones made from real hair, and they were about 10 percent of the cost.

Wigs for Church, and Hats for Every Day. I ended up using hats for my everyday look and to wear for work. Just as with my wardrobe, I found my favorite hat at a thrift store. In addition, I found hats at garage sales, department stores, and TLC (Tender Loving Care, a website and catalog of the American Cancer Society). And I received many hats as gifts from friends and other cancer survivors.

My misguided assumption was that my favorite hat would turn out to be one with a large, floppy brim. Boy was I wrong! Reality proved to be the complete opposite. I didn't wear one. I felt vulnerable and lived in fear that the Illinois wind could catch it and blow it off my head. I was open with my battle with cancer, but not that open. I preferred wearing hats that I knew had a more likely chance of staying on my head throughout the day.

Note: Hats did not make my head as uncomfortable and itchy as wigs. For some reason I avoided using scarves, but the American Cancer Society has great tips to help survivors get acquainted with their various uses.

Symmetry is Overrated

ME

I am providing the following information simply to share my perspective. Surgical options are an extremely personal choice. But sometimes it is good to receive feedback from someone who has already traveled the same path.

One Scoop, Sundae or a Banana Split. Making the choice regarding surgery proved to be the most difficult for me. It did not help that I was having to make irreversible decisions while on the tails of hearing the word cancer and my name in the same sentence. The surgeons gave me the options of a lumpectomy, single mastectomy, or a double. Even though it was only two weeks from official diagnosis to surgery, the process seemed like it took forever. There was this sense of urgency to get things done quickly. I was obsessed with the fact that there was cancer in me. I wanted to get it out! But I had to keep in mind this was a big decision that I could not reverse. My first instinct was to take them both with no reconstruction. After talking it over with my family, my husband, and my support group, I ended up choosing a single mastectomy with no reconstruction.

Got a Sneak Peek of Life on the Other Side. I visited the store that matched me with the prosthesis I would use after surgery. The clerk was happy to show me one, and I was able to touch it and see how heavy it was. It took the unknown factor away from me. I now knew what to expect before I made a decision not to do reconstruction. She also showed me a post-surgery bra that helped tremendously, which I purchased before my surgery.

I also browsed around the bra section and found comfort knowing they sold bras similar to ones I enjoyed using in the past. The only difference was that these had pockets in which to secure the prosthesis.

After about a year I asked my mother-in-law if she could sew a pocket onto one of my favorite bras from my pre-surgery days. She did, and I loved it. She created her own design, and it worked great. There are catalogs, however, like TLC, that sell prefabricated pockets that may be sewn into a conventional bra.

Another favorite of mine is a mastectomy bra with lace that comes up pretty high in the cleavage area. This lacey, modesty panel hides the scar well and allows me to wear more fashionable, lower-cut apparel.

Binky and Boo. Strangely enough these were my husband's pet names for my breasts years before the mastectomy. Maybe it was God's way of preparing us for this chapter of our lives, because they already had names that were suitable for after surgery – one with a nipple, named Binky, and one, a ghost, named Boo.

At first I felt like a freak with just one breast. But after the initial shock, I changed my mindset to being thankful I still had one breast. If they had taken both, I wouldn't again experience what that special feeling adds during intimacy.

My husband is an angel. There isn't a day that goes by that he does not tell me how beautiful I am, especially when I am without my prosthesis. He was 100 percent supportive of my decision for a mastectomy without reconstruction.

Another consideration for keeping Binky was my active lifestyle. I figured if I had one breast it would keep my prosthesis in place and anchor my bra down. Without one secure breast I envisioned lifting both arms to block a volleyball during a game and having to pull both my breasts back down into place. I'm not sure of my assumption, but I wanted no part of that.

Misconceptions about Chemotherapy

ME

I struggled with where to insert this information, but decided all this was more about my spirit than the experience. There were so many aspects of cancer treatment that frankly terrified me, but it was nothing like what I imagined. So, I decided to take a moment to share my misconceptions and pleasant surprises about chemotherapy, ports, post-surgical fears, and the benefits of a second opinion.

Chemotherapy. Although each treatment wrote its own history, there were also similarities. For instance, on the third day after every treatment, my energy was sluggish, and my appetite was lighter than normal. But after every infusion, I felt like me again by the sixth day. On day seven I returned to work for the next two weeks. So, there were some consistencies with the treatments that allowed me to plan.

The side effects of each treatment, however, were all very different. That is the part that surprised me. I am not sharing this information to suggest that everyone will have similar outcomes. But I list my experiences to illustrate that there is definitely a component of chemotherapy that can be unpredictable. To the best of my recollection, here is what I remember:

- *First treatment:* There was discomfort in my abdomen by my liver (acute at times; I contemplated going to the emergency room), bowel issues (including diarrhea and green stools with strange masses in them), mild mouth sores. Within two weeks my hair was gone.
- *Second treatment:* My feet were peeling, and the second toe on my right foot was numb.
- *Third treatment:* My hands peeled (I found relief by washing them in cold water rather than hot), and more of my toes were becoming numb.
- *Fourth treatment:* There was nothing new, but all my toes were numb and tingling.
- *Fifth treatment:* I fainted one evening; afterward my temperature reading was 94 degrees.
- *Sixth treatment:* Again, there was nothing new, and I was done with the initial round of chemotherapy except for Herceptin.
- *Post treatment:* My eyebrows fell out, but my hair started to grow everywhere else. Yes, they fell out after I was done with treatment. I have talked to other survivors who had the same experience; it was not what we expected.
- *What treatment was not:* It did not make me vomit, frail, or bedridden.

I anticipated chemotherapy to be a lot worse than it was. I never took a trip to my primary care physician or the emergency room during treatment. I share all this because I had the misconception that each treatment would be relatively the same—which they were in some respects, but not all.

Ports, They Sounded Scary to Me. Ports are simply a way to allow the doctor more easy access to one of the larger vessels in our circulatory system for the administration of chemotherapy drugs. The way I understand it is if doctors use the veins in our arms, after time they may become damaged. Since chemotherapy is so caustic, it is typically dispersed more effectively where there is a greater blood supply.

I thought ports were outside the body like those used for dialysis patients. I was relieved to know that ports for chemotherapy are usually under the skin. I envisioned my chest like a gas cap on my car, as they filled me up every three weeks. I was relieved to discover it was more discreet than I predicted.

I continued life as normally as I did before the port was inserted. I played volleyball, enjoyed inner-tubing behind the boat and rode the attractions at amusement parks. I still ride roller coasters, but I have bowed out of riding super, intense roller coasters, since the security harness comes down directly over my port. But I figure that is not a huge sacrifice!

I am thankful I have the port. It could have been a tough road without it. The veins in my arms are already worn out from giving so much blood; I can't imagine trying to put well over sixty infusions through them too.

Note: It was a couple months before I could sleep on my side again, but eventually I rarely even notice the port existed.

Post-Surgery Tips that May Help. When I went out in public, I found it helpful to use one of those rock-climbing clips to attach the post-surgery drain up by where my breast used to be. When I coupled this technique with loose-fitting clothing, it hid my chest's lack of symmetry and concealed the drain. I didn't let a drain keep me at home.

Speaking of drains, I lost sleep over worrying about the removal of the drainage tubes. When I was a young adult, I listened while my own mother's tubes were removed from her chest cavity after a major car accident. Her screams of pain were etched into my memory, and they fueled the anxiety of the impending removal of my own tubes. Fortunately, my experience was nothing like my mother's was years earlier. When the doctors removed my drains, it felt like butterflies flew from my chest. I was so relieved, but so disappointed I spent all that time worrying over something that merely tickled.

Consider a Second Opinion. Chemotherapy can be scary in the beginning. I believed that I had a better chance of survival if I truly believed I made the right decision. So I sought a second opinion. Hearing that both doctors agreed on the same plan of attack put my mind more at ease. The second opinion helped me not second-guess my choice of treatment.

The oncologist who provided the second opinion also explained the discomfort I was experiencing. I had a lot of pain in the side where my liver is located. I thought the worst, of course. She told me the pain may be a good sign. Whenever the tumors are destroyed, the liver regenerates in the pockets where the masses formerly were. This can cause aches. From that point on, the pain brought me joy instead of fear. I was thankful that her expertise not only provided peace of mind, but also an uplifting perspective.

Note: Try to not let the expense inhibit you from obtaining the knowledge of another oncologist. The cost of attaining at least one other opinion is covered by most insurance companies. I personally did not pay anything out of pocket to receive this advice. I believe that, when receiving a second opinion, you should consider going to a hospital known for cancer treatment and research, but which your current oncologist has no affiliation with, so that you receive a fresh, unprejudiced perspective.

Conclusion

The best way I can sum up this journey is to compare it to an experience I had years earlier at the Brickyard in Indianapolis. I had an opportunity to attend a stock car race. I was far from a Nascar fan but I was invited to go. The beginning of the race was intense as the military jets flew overhead; it was shortly after the events of September 11th. I shed uncontrollable tears, as I could not recall a time of such moving and spiritual patriotism in my life.

The end of the race was also sensational as we waited in eager anticipation of seeing who came out victorious. It was just the middle of the race I struggled with. I had a hard time staying interested in watching the cars continually jockey for position. So I started studying the people in the stands. I distinctly remember seeing a beach ball out there over the crowd. It stayed up in the air for what seemed like hours. It was briefly touched by one person and sent off to the next.

This is the most down-to-earth analogy I can use to describe how people have influenced me. I truly believe that they were placed by God to help guide me. Their impact may have only lasted a moment, but all these encounters added up to something that kept me aloft, just like that beach ball.

It is scripture, however, that provides the most suitable closing. I could not have written it for you better myself. Ephesians 3:14-21 (NLT), Paul's prayer for spiritual growth reads:

When I think of all this, I fall to my knees and pray to the Father, the Creator of everything in heaven and on earth. I pray that from his glorious, unlimited resources he will empower you with inner strength through his Spirit. Then Christ will make his home in your hearts as you trust in him. Your roots will grow down into God's love and keep you strong. And may you have the power to understand, as all God's people should, how wide, how long, how high, and how deep his love is. May you experience the love of Christ, though it is too great to understand fully. Then you will be made complete with all the fullness of life and power that comes from God. Now all glory to God, who is able, through his mighty power at work within us, to accomplish infinitely more than we might ask or think. Glory to him in the church and in Christ Jesus through all generations forever and ever! Amen.

Bibliography

Chapter 1: The Choice is Ultimately Ours

Environmental Working Group (website). Accessed July 13, 2014. http://www.ewg.org/foodnews.

http://www.ams.usda.gov/AMSv1.0/getfile?dDocName=STLDEV3004446&acct=nopgeninfo USDA, National Organic Program (pdf file online). Publication date October 2012. Accessed November 17, 2013.

Malkmus, George, Peter Shockey, and Stowe Shockey. *The Hallelujah Diet*. Shippensburg: Destiny Image Publishers, Inc., 2006.

Campbell, T. Colin, PhD., and Thomas M Campbell II. *The China Study*. Dallas: BenBella Books, Inc., 2006.

Cohen, Alissa and Leah Dubois. *Raw Food for Everyone*. New York: Penguin Group, 2010.

Rubin, Jordan S. *The Maker's Diet*. Lake Mary: Siloam, 2004, 2005.

Dr. Peter J. D'Adamo and Catherine Whitney. *Live Right 4 Your Type*. New York: G. P. Putnum's Sons, 2001.

USDA, Xianli Wu, Gary R. Beecher, Joanne M. Holden, David B. Haytowitz, Susan E. Gebhardt, and Ronald L. Prior. "Lipophilic Properties of Antioxidants." http://longevity.about.com/od/lifelongnutrition/a/antioxidants.htm Publication date 2004. Accessed December 2013 on About.com.

http://www.holisticonline.com/Remedies/hrt/hrt_food_and_estrogen.htm Holistic Online (website). Accessed December 14, 2013.

http://www.nlm.nih.gov/m/pubmed PubMed (Website). Accessed March 13, 2014.

Colbert, MD, Don. *The Seven Pillars of Health*. Lake Mary: Siloam, 2007.

Shinya, MD, Hiromi. *The Enzyme Factor*. Originally published in Japanese by Sunmark Press, First English-language edition, third printing 2009.

Chapter 2: External Influences Utilizing Complementary and Alternative Therapies

Colbert, MD, Don. *The New Bible Cure for Cancer A Dietary Answer*. Lake Mary: Siloam, 2010.

Ober, Clinton, Stephen T Sinatra, M.D., and Martin Zucker. *Earthing: The most important health discovery ever?*. Laguna Beach: Basic Health Publications, Inc., 2010.

Chapter 3: Rebuilding Spirit From Within

Anderson, Greg. *Cancer: 50 Essential Things to Do*. New York: Penguin Group, 2009.

Chapter 4: A Light That Breaks Forth Like the Dawn

Melander, Rochelle. *Write-A-Thon*. Cincinnati: Writer's Digest Books, 2011.

Rubin, Gretchen. *The Happiness Project*. New York: HarperCollins Publishers, 2009.

Wertich, Laurie. "Friends through Thick and Thin." Cancer Fighters Thrive Spring 2012: 22-25.

Rate and Monitor Your Results

Copy this page for each section you try
On a scale of 1-10, with 10 being the highest,
rate how the lifestyle change transformed the quality of your life.

Topic:____

Should I consider seeking doctor approval first? Yes No

Energy	1 2 3 4 5 6 7 8 9 10
Digestion / Elimination	1 2 3 4 5 6 7 8 9 10
Sleep Quality	1 2 3 4 5 6 7 8 9 10
Spirit/Happiness	1 2 3 4 5 6 7 8 9 10
Stress Management	1 2 3 4 5 6 7 8 9 10
Weight	1 2 3 4 5 6 7 8 9 10
Muscle, Joint pain	1 2 3 4 5 6 7 8 9 10
Worth the time	1 2 3 4 5 6 7 8 9 10
Cost worth the results	1 2 3 4 5 6 7 8 9 10

Total Points: ___________

Note: Use the back of the page to record notes about your experience after trying these lifestyle changes, or utilize the space to document publications that provided additional guidance. It is not exclusively about assigning a value to something, but chances are the items with higher point values will provide a greater benefit. Express how it changed your life for better or worse. Documentation may help you recall the experience, which will not only benefit you, but possibly support others.

When doing further research, try to abide by the five-click rule for internet searches. If you do not find what you want in five clicks, get out and move on. Tear out magazine articles rather than keeping the whole periodical. And consider using a scanner, so you can copy pages from books that interest you rather than having to look them up when needed for future reference.

Cancer Timeline

(October 2009 to December 2013)

October 2009

- Felt a small pea sized lump in my breast.
- Went for my annual gynecological appointment. No further testing was done.

November 2009 - February 2010

- Life happened. I forgot about checking the lump for progression. Thinking cancer can't happen to me! It does not even run in our family.
- By the time I checked it again in February it was about 1 centimeter. We were on vacation in Mexico.

April 2010

- Core biopsy confirmed the mass in my left breast was cancerous. I was 41.
- The first book I bought was The Bible.
- I immediately changed my diet. The second book I purchased was *The Maker's Diet,* discussed in the nutrition chapter.
- Pathology revealed the tumor was triple positive, meaning the tumor had estrogen, progesterone and HER2 receptors. The HER2 component was not confirmed until further FISH testing was performed.
- The doctors left the decision for lumpectomy, single radical mastectomy or a double mastectomy up to me.

May 2010

- After an MRI to determine the chances of disease in my right breast, I chose a radical mastectomy of my left breast and opted for no reconstruction.
    - • The surgery went very well by most standards.
    - • There were good margins—meaning there were no cancerous cells in the tissues surrounding the tumor.
    - • There was no lymph node involvement; they were free of cancer cells.
    - • I experienced a very typical recovery without any complications.
- After the surgery, I was officially diagnosed as a stage II breast cancer patient. Stage II because size of the tumor was between 2 to 5 centimeters (it measured 3.5 by 2.0 by 1.7 centimeters), and because no cancer was detected in the lymph nodes.

• The pathology report from the surgery read, "positive for residual infiltrating ductal carcinoma and ductal carcinoma in situ."

June 2010

• I was experiencing discomfort in my abdomen; a PET scan revealed there were cancerous lesions on my liver. I was now Stage IV.
• I decided which clinic I would receive treatment from.
• A CAT scan revealed there were also multiple growths in both lungs.
  - • Surgery was not an option because the liver and lungs had multiple masses.
  - • There were numerous ill-defined hypodense masses in both lobes of the liver that were documented by the CAT scan, one recorded at 2.5 by 3.8 centimeters and another at 3.7 by 3.9 centimeters. The largest left lobe lesion was 1.5 centimeters.
  - • The CAT scan also revealed numerous 0.8 centimeter or smaller non-calcified nodules throughout both lungs.
  - • The results from a bone scan documented an area in my sternum that was questionably cancer, but it was not confirmed by further testing.
  - • A brain scan was also ordered, but no disease was found.

• I received a second opinion from another doctor at a different medical center. She agreed with the treatment plan that the first doctor had recommended for me.

June 2010 – October 2010

• Chemotherapy started: Herceptin, Taxotere and Cytoxan every three weeks.
• The treatment during chemotherapy also included a Lupron shot every three months to keep my ovaries dormant.
• I continued with a good nutritional regimen. Once I was done with the Maker's Diet (a forty-day eating plan), I incorporated the Blood-Type Diet by Dr. D'Adamo.
• Walking was my preferred choice for exercise. I also played volleyball.
• I added many alternative therapies, which are discussed throughout the book, such as massage, chiropractic, and acupuncture.

November 2010

• The first scans taken after the first round of chemotherapy showed no evidence of disease. Furthermore, no evidence of disease was found in my blood work.
• Taxotere and Cytoxan were removed from my treatment plan.
• I remained on Herceptin and the Lupron shot.
• Tamoxifen was added; this is a pill that is taken daily to reduce my estrogen.

March 2011

• Another PET and CAT scan was ordered. There was still no evidence of disease.
• The team of doctors monitoring my care used the word remission. I experienced a progression from stage IV breast cancer to remission in nine months. I considered it a rebirth—a second chance.

April 2011

- Walked a half marathon in under four hours.

May 2011-March 2013

Continued with Herceptin, Lupron and Tamoxifen.

April 2013-November 2013

- Lupron was removed; Down to just Herceptin and Tamoxifen.

December 2013

- Only on Tamoxifen.
- Remind myself that worry serves no purpose.
- And thankful every day for how the grace of God works in my life.

Christine's Stay Disease-Free Plan

I have a close friend who was diagnosed with advanced stage ovarian cancer a couple years after I was diagnosed with breast cancer. We attended a gathering with mutual friends, and I had an opportunity to give her aspects of coping with cancer that seemed to work well for me. The atmosphere was not conducive to sharing a lot of details, but I offered some general guidelines. I recall telling her the importance of nutrition, exercise and relieving stress. In essence I gave her fifteen minutes of basics, and she took it from there. Her plan is listed below. She was diagnosed in May of 2012, and as of 2014, she was experiencing a remarkable quality of life. I share this list, with her permission, to illustrate the commonality of how she adapted to her life with cancer and how it generally parallels the information that I just shared in the proceeding pages. Because, although there was a common thread, there was also a flair that was just hers because she created her own plan.

Note: Her surgery lasted all day. This was not a textbook case of ovarian cancer.

Nutrition

Eat Slowly!!

<u>Food – Yes (at least 80 percent)</u>

- Unlimited fresh vegetables (organic or washed thoroughly)
- *daily:* kale, spinach, broccoli, cabbage
- fresh fruit – bright colored (berries daily)
- organic raw nuts, seeds, unsweetened dried fruit/coconut
- free range poultry & eggs
- wild caught fish & seafood
- olive oil, coconut oil, organic spices
- green tea (2 cups daily)
- filtered/spring water (3-5 glasses daily)
- grass fed dairy or raw dairy, butter, ghee (limited)
- organic whole grains & legumes (limited)
- grass fed beef & pork (limited)

<u>Food – Avoid! (Less than 20 percent)</u>

- everything processed in a bag or box
- refined flour & other grains, pasta, rice, cereals
- sugar or anything with added sugar, desserts

- fast food, lunch meat, processed cheese
- pop, alcohol, sweetened beverages, diet pop
- corn oil, all vegetable oils, margarine, etc.
- stimulants, caffeine
- artificial sweeteners, preservatives, etc.

Exercise

- strength/interval training (2–3 times a week)
- walking/low impact light cardio (5–7 times a week)
- stretching or yoga (daily)
- spend time outdoors as much as possible

Stress relief & relaxation

- breathing exercises (2 times daily)
- mindful meditation, positive affirmations (30 minutes 4-7 times a week)
- get up from desk/sitting every 30 min and move/stretch
- spend more time with friends/family or talking with friends/family
- Go to bed and wake up at the same time every day & get 8 hours of sleep
- spend time outdoors as much as possible
- spend more me time
- Eat slowly!!!!!

Supplements

- good multivitamin with minerals (daily as directed)
- fish oil (5 times a day)
- Circumin (2 times a day)
- probiotics (daily)
- Mushroom complex (daily)
- vitamin D (daily)
- melatonin (20 mg daily)

Miscellaneous stuff

- threw out all plastic microwave containers
- replace all non-stick pans with stainless steel
- slowly getting all natural cleaning products
- all natural toothpaste
- body care without parabens, etc.
- get more plants
- have a bigger garden

Other Organizations That Helped

Organizations that helped our entire family:

MEMORIES OF LOVE
www.memoriesoflove.org

They help create lasting and loving memories by sending the entire family for five days to Orlando, Florida, for a fun-filled vacation far removed from mounting medical bills, therapy, and hospital visits. Through the generosity of corporate partners and sponsors, they are able to provide tickets to the area's best-loved theme parks: Universal Studios/Island of Adventures and Sea World, as well as a beautiful room at one of a number of Orlando/Kissimmee Resorts, discount meal vouchers, and financial support for travel and incidentals.

LITTLE PINK HOUSES OF HOPE
www.littlepink.org

They provide FREE week-long vacations for breast cancer patients and their families. They believe a cancer diagnosis does not just affect the patient, but the entire family. Every beach retreat is designed to help families relax, reconnect, and rejuvenate during the cancer journey.

Organizations that helped me:

BREAST CANCER RECOVERY
www.bcrecovery.org

Breast Cancer Recovery's mission is to provide environments for women breast cancer survivors to heal emotionally. All programs are designed and conducted by survivors for survivors. They offer wellness retreats—Infinite Boundaries—for women in all stages of breast cancer: newly diagnosed, in treatment, and many years finished with treatment. Women ages twenty-one to eighty have attended their retreats.

IMERMAN ANGELS
www.imermanangels.org

Imerman Angels provides personalized connections that enable one-on-one support among cancer fighters, survivors, and caregivers. All services are free and provided for any type, age, and stage of cancer.

YOUNG SURVIVAL COALITION
www.youngsurvival.org

Young Survival Coalition (YSC) is the premier global organization dedicated to the critical issues unique to young women who are diagnosed with breast cancer. YSC offers resources, connections, and outreach, so women feel supported, empowered, and hopeful.

(All websites referenced were accessed in December of 2013.)